PTCB SIMPLIFIED

PHARMACY TECHNICIAN CERTIFICATION EXAM STUDY GUIDE

— 2ND EDITION —

BY
DAVID A HECKMAN, PHARMD

www.RxStudyGuides.com
Be Prepared and Confident on Exam Day

PTCB® Exam Simplified
Pharmacy Technician Certification Exam Study Guide
2ND Edition

ISBN-13: 978-1942682011
ISBN-10: 1942682018

PTCB® is a registered trademark of the Pharmacy Technician Certification Board. The Pharmacy Technician Certification Board does not endorse or promote this or any other PTCB® exam study guide.

The author does not assume and hereby disclaims any liability to any party for losses, damages, and/or failures resulting from an error or omission, regardless of cause.

This publication is not a substitute for legal advice. For legal advice, consult a legal professional.

This publication does not contain actual exam questions.

Book cover design by **Keeling Design & Media, Inc.**

Published by Heckman Media

Printed in the United States of America

A study guide for the *updated* Pharmacy Technician Certification Exam

The Pharmacy Technician Certification Board announced that the certification exam has been reorganized into the following 9 knowledge domains as of November 1st, 2013:

1. Pharmacology for Technicians (13.75%)
2. Pharmacy Law and Regulations (12.5%)
3. Sterile and Non-sterile Compounding (8.75%)
4. Medication Safety (12.5%)
5. Pharmacy Quality Assurance (7.5%)
6. Medication Order Entry and Fill Process (17.5%)
7. Pharmacy Inventory Management (8.75%)
8. Pharmacy Billing and Reimbursement (8.75%)
9. Pharmacy Information Systems Usage and Application (10%)

This study guide provides a review of the most important information from the 9 knowledge domains that comprise the PTCB® exam. To facilitate and expedite the learning process, the content is presented in a format that allows you to test yourself as you study. Once you are familiar with the content of this study guide, use a note card or piece of paper to cover up the answers and quiz yourself. Good luck!

- $129 exam registration fee
- Administered at Pearson Vue testing centers
- Computer-based exam
- 90 multiple-choice questions
- Basic calculator provided
- No penalties for guessing
- 120 minutes to complete
    - 5 minute introductory tutorial
    - 110 minute examination
    - 5 minute exit survey
- Score range: 300 – 900
    - Must achieve a score of 650 or higher to pass
        - Answer ~ 70% of questions correct to score 650

First Order of Business
Get You Up To Speed

Before we delve into the material you are likely to see on the PTCB exam, we need to review some basic pharmacy topics. This portion of the study guide will be especially helpful for those of you who have little to no prior experience working in pharmacy. First, we will review what pharmacy practice is and talk about the sort of functions you will and will not perform as a pharmacy technician. Then we will talk about the different types of drug companies and the various types of drug names (brand/trade names, generic names, and chemical names). Next, we will review basic mathematical proportions – an extremely important problem-solving tool that you will use on the PTCB exam and every day as a pharmacy technician. And finally, before proceeding to the main content of the study guide, we will review key terms.

When you look at the official PTCB exam blueprint (available at www.ptcb.org), you will see that math is a huge part of the exam. To give yourself the best chance of passing, you need to become an expert in pharmacy math. This study guide with help you obtain that expertise by guiding you through numerous examples and providing several practice problems. Another area you should focus on is pharmacy law and regulations. Pharmacy is one of the most heavily regulated professions. With so many potential issues involving ethics, safety, and privacy this comes as no surprise. Be prepared and know the pertinent laws and regulations well. While reviewing each topic on the PTCB exam blueprint is important in preparation for the PTCB exam, a working knowledge of pharmacy math and pharmacy law – along with brand and generic drug names – provides the basic foundation that every technician needs to be successful. Keep this in mind as you prepare for your career as a certified pharmacy technician.

What major activities fall under the scope of pharmacy practice?
- Interpreting, evaluating, and implementing medical & prescription orders.
- Compounding & dispensing prescriptions.
- Participating in the selection and administration of drugs and medical devices.
- Performing drug utilization reviews.
- Maintaining patient medication profiles and pharmacy records.
- Counseling patients.
- Administering vaccinations/immunizations.
- Performing drug-related research.

Certain functions may only be performed by a licensed pharmacist. What are some examples?
- Evaluating prescriptions for conformance with legal requirements, authenticity, accuracy, and interactions with other drugs.
- Making determinations of therapeutic equivalency.
- Performing drug utilization reviews.
- Signing or initialing a record of dispensing.
- Counseling patients.
- Performing functions that require professional judgment.
- Administering vaccinations/immunizations.

What are some common functions that pharmacy technicians are typically authorized to perform?
- Creating & maintaining patient medication profiles and pharmacy records.
- Receiving written or electronically transmitted prescriptions.
- Typing prescription labels.
- Filling prescription orders.
  - Retrieving drugs from stock.
  - Counting dosage units.
  - Placing dosage units in a container.
  - Affixing a label to the container.
  - Returning drugs to stock.
- Handling or delivering completed prescriptions.
- Alerting the pharmacist to potential issues/problems.
- Maintaining organization in the pharmacy.

There are two types of drug companies - <u>innovator</u> drug companies and <u>generic</u> drug companies. Innovator drug companies are heavily involved in drug discovery research and clinical trials to determine the safety and effectiveness of potential new drugs. Discovering a new drug that is both safe and effective is a challenging task. The chance of one new drug making it to market is less than one-tenth of one percent! When a new drug is discovered, the drug company files a patent for the drug and then attempts to prove that the drug is safe and effective so FDA approval can be obtained. Drug patents are good for about 20 years. The company that discovers a new drug gets the exclusive right to manufacture it (no other drug company can copy their idea) until the patent on the drug expires. Companies generally file the patent before clinical trials begin. It typically takes 10 to 13 years for a drug to obtain FDA approval after it has been discovered (that is, *if* it gains FDA approval). For this reason, when most new drugs finally reach the market, the innovator company typically only gets 7 to 10 years of exclusive manufacturing rights, as this is all the time that remains on the patent. Innovator drug companies typically charge a high price for new drugs because they need to recuperate the expenses that have accumulated from years of research and development and still turn a profit. Once the patent expires, generic drug companies start selling their own copy of the drug. Since generic drug companies do not have nearly as many research and development expenses, they can charge a much lower price than the innovator drug company. Oftentimes, innovator drug companies hire lawyers to find ways to acquire patent term extensions, so it is very difficult to predict exactly when a brand name drug will become available generically.

Examples of Innovator Drug Companies:

Merck & Co.	GlaxoSmithKline	Sanofi
Johnson & Johnson	Abbott	Atrazeneca
Eli Lilly	Amgen	
Pfizer	Roche	

Examples of Generic Drug Companies:

Mylan	Watson	Dr. Reddy's
Actavis	Greenstone	Mallinckrodt
TEVA	Hospira	Lupin
Sandoz	Apotex	Par

You will be expected to know both the generic name for a brand name drug and vice versa. Brand names and generic names are often used interchangeably by patients and healthcare professionals, so it is important that you know both names.

Every drug has a chemical name, a generic name, and a brand name. There is a lot going on here; how do you keep it all straight? Let's break it down:

Chemical Names – The chemical name of a drug is rarely ever used in pharmacy. Chemical names are assigned using a naming system developed by the International Union of Pure and Applied Chemistry (IUPAC). Although the naming system may seem complicated, it simply names molecules based on their chemical structure. One chemical name most people are familiar with is "ethanol," the type of alcohol found in alcoholic beverages. The name, ethanol comes from "ethane," which is the IUPAC name for a molecule made up of 2 carbon atoms. The "–ol" suffix is the IUPAC suffix used to indicate that an alcohol (-OH) group is attached to the molecule. Chemical drug names are assigned using this same type of scientific naming system (no creativity involved whatsoever!). For instance, the chemical name of the active ingredient in Tylenol® (generic name: acetaminophen) is N-acetyl-p-aminophenol. If you have ever heard acetaminophen abbreviated as APAP, this is where that abbreviation comes from (N-acetyl-p-aminophenol). As mentioned previously, the chemical name of a drug is rarely, if ever, used in pharmacy, but generic names and brand names are used commonly.

Generic Names – In the United States of America, generic names are assigned by the United States Adopted Names Council (USAN). The USAN prevents a new drug from being given a name that is similar to a drug that is already available on the market. It is important that drug names be unique to prevent mistakes by prescribers and misinterpretation of prescription orders by pharmacists and pharmacy technicians. A synonym for "generic name" is "established name."

Brand Names – A brand name is assigned to a drug by the company that discovered the drug (the innovator drug company). During the time when the drug is under patent, the drug is only produced by the innovator drug company using the brand name. After the patent expires, the drug may still be available in the brand name form from the innovator drug company, but it will also be available under its generic name from one or more generic manufacturers. Some drug companies may create a new brand name for their version of the generically available drug. This is why we sometimes see drugs with two or more brand names. Synonyms for "brand name" include "trade name" and "proprietary name."

Most of the math you will face on the PTCB exam involves proportions. The following is an example of a proportion:

$$\frac{a}{b} = \frac{c}{d}$$

When you get a proportion problem, you must first cross multiply. For example:

$$\frac{a}{b} = \frac{c}{d} \quad \therefore \quad a \times d = b \times c$$

Then isolate the unknown. For instance:

$$a = \frac{b \times c}{d} \quad \text{or} \quad b = \frac{a \times d}{c} \quad \text{or} \quad c = \frac{a \times d}{b} \quad \text{or} \quad d = \frac{b \times c}{a}$$

Here is an example of a real-life problem that involves proportions:
A car travels at a speed of 60 miles per hour. How many miles does the car travel in 2.5 hours?

$$\frac{60 \text{ miles}}{1 \text{ hour}} = \frac{\chi \text{ miles}}{2.5 \text{ hours}} \quad \therefore \quad \chi \text{ miles} = \frac{60 \text{ miles} \times 2.5 \text{ hours}}{1 \text{ hour}} = 150 \text{ miles}$$

Be sure that the units match on each side of the proportion. For instance, let's say the question was: how many miles were traveled in 150 <u>minutes</u>?

To solve this problem, you would first need to convert the units from minutes to hours like this:

$$150 \text{ minutes} \times \frac{1 \text{ hour}}{60 \text{ minutes}} = 2.5 \text{ hours}$$

Notice how the units cancel out.

The same approach can be used for solving problems in pharmacy. For instance, let's say you are dispesnsing 50 tablets to a patient that is taking 2 tablets per day. How many days will the bottle of 50 tablets last?

$$50 \text{ tablets} \times \frac{\text{day}}{2 \text{ tablets}} = 25 \text{ days}$$

The term 1 hour/60 minutes is a "conversion factor." When we multiplied 150 minutes by 1hour/60 minutes, we essentially multiplied the value 150 minutes by a factor of 1. Why? Because this calculation did not increase or decrease the amount of time the car was traveling; it just changed the units used to express the amount of time traveled (150 minutes and 2.5 hours are the same amount of time). You will be using conversion factors frequently when solving pharmacy math problems. For instance, one conversion factor commonly used in pharmacy is 5 milliliters/1 teaspoonful (can also be expressed as 1 teaspoonful/5 milliliters). You need to memorize this conversion factor and a few others (see the list of **Must-Know Conversion Factors** in the section titled "The Secret to Solving Nearly Any Pharmacy Math Problem").

Most medical terms are composed of Greek or Latin prefixes, root words, and/or suffixes. For this reason, we will use the next few pages to study and learn the most common Greek and Latin prefixes, root words, and suffixes seen in medical terms.

Prefix, Root, or Suffix	Meaning	Example
-al	Pertaining to	Abdominal
Angi(o)-	Blood vessel	Angioedema
Ante-	Before	Ante room
Anti-	Against/opposed to	Antivenom
Arthr(o)-	Pertaining to joints	Arthritis
Bio-	Life	Biohazard
Brady-	Abnormally slow	Bradycardia
Bucc(o)-	Cheek	Buccal
-cardi(o)-	Heart	Cardiology
Centi-	Hundred	Centimeter
Derm(o)-	Skin	Dermatology
-emesis	Vomiting	Hyperemesis
-emia	Blood	Hyperkalemia
-glyc(o)-	Sugar	Hyperglycemic
Heter(o)-	Different	Heterogenous
Hom(o)-	The same	Homogenous
Hyper-	Beyond normal	Hypertension
Hyp(o)-	Below normal	Hypoglycemia
-ic	Pertaining to	Gastric bypass
-ism	Condition/ disease	Hypothyroidism
-itis	Inflammation	Nephritis
-kal-	Potassium	Hypokalemia
Kilo-	Thousand	Kilogram
Lacrim(o)-	Tear	Lacrimation
-logy	The study of	Biology
Micro-	Millionth	Microgram
Milli-	Thousandth	Milligram
Nas(o)-	Pertaining to the nose	Nasal Spray
-oma	Mass/tumor	Sarcoma
Ophthalm(o)-	Pertaining to the eye	Ophthalmology
-osis	Condition/disease	Diverticulosis
Ot(o)-	Pertaining to the ear	Otic
-penia	Deficiency	Osteopenia

Prefix, Root, or Suffix	Meaning	Example
Pharmaco-	Drug	Pharmacology
Poly–	Many/several	Polyuria
Post–	After	Postpartum
Pyr(o)-	Fever	Antipyretic
Ren(o)-	Kidneys	Renal function
-stasis	Standing/stopping	Hemostasis
-staxis	Dripping	Epistaxis
Tachy–	Abnormally fast	Tachycardia
-tension/-tensive	Pressure	Hypertension
Thromb(o)-	Related to the clotting of blood	Thrombosis
-uric(o)-	Uric acid	Hyperuricemia
-ur(o)-	Pertaining to urine	Nocturia

Absorption – the movement of a drug from a delivery medium (e.g. tablet, capsule, trandermal patch) into the bloodstream.

Agonist – a substance that stimulates an action. For example, stimulation of beta-1 receptors results in an elevated heart rate. The body naturally produces adrenaline (or "epinephrine") to stimulate these receptors and achieve this effect; therefore, adrenaline is an agonist. There are also several drugs that act as beta-1 receptor agonists (e.g. dobutamine, isoproterenol, EpiPen®).

Angina – severe chest pain caused by insufficient blood flow to the heart.

Antagonist – a substance that opposes an action. For example, metoprolol is a beta-1 receptor antagonist (more commonly known as a "beta blocker"). Metoprolol opposes the stimulation of beta-1 receptors, thus suppressing the heart rate.

Ante area – the space directly adjacent to the clean room. The air quality in the ante area should be at least ISO class 8 (see the term "ISO classification" for more details).

Antitussive – an agent used to suppress a cough. Antitussives are a particularly good choice for patients that have a nonproductive cough.

Arteries – the blood vessels that carry blood from the heart to the organs.

Atrial fibrillation – a type of cardiac arrhythmia in which the right atrium (the top right portion of the heart) receives irregular electrical impulses from the nervous system causing the heart to beat too rapidly. People with atrial fibrillation are at an increased risk of stroke because the irregular heartbeat can lead to the formation of a blood clot that is capable of traveling to the brain. Sometimes atrial fibrillation is referred to as "AF" or "A-fib." Atrial fibrillation is the most common type of cardiac arrhythmia.

Benign prostatic hyperplasia (BPH) – a non-cancerous condition in which the prostate gland is enlarged. The enlarged prostate presses against the urethra, blocking urinary outflow. Only men can get BPH because only men have a prostate gland.

Blood glucose – a measure of the concentration of glucose (sugar) in the blood. High blood glucose is a sign of diabetes.

Blood clot – a mass of coagulated blood.

Bradycardia – below normal heart rate at rest. (Normal resting heart rate is 60-90 beats per minute.)

Cardiac arrhythmia – any condition in which the heart does not beat regularly (e.g. beats off rhythm, beats too fast, beats too slow). Other terms for cardiac arrhythmia include "cardiac dysrhythmia" and "irregular heartbeat."

Cardiovascular system – the organ system composed of the heart and the blood vessels (arteries and veins).

Ceiling effect – the therapeutic effect increases only up to a certain point (the "ceiling"). Higher doses impart no additional benefit and do more harm than good, causing more side effects without increasing the therapeutic effect.

Clean room – The room/area designated for sterile compounding. A clean room may also be referred to as a "buffer area." The air quality in a clean room should be at least ISO class 7.

Clostridium difficile – a species of bacteria that can infect the intestines and cause a serious condition called pseudomembranous colitis. Pseudomembranous colitis is characterized by severe diarrhea, fever, and abdominal pain which can lead to dehydration, electrolyte imbalances, and in some cases death. Clostridium difficile can be abrreviated as C. difficile or C. diff. Most antibiotic drugs promote infection of the intestine by C. difficile (a rare but very serious risk of antibiotic use). When antibiotics are used to kill bacteria causing some type of infection (e.g. a sinus infection), they also end up killing a portion of the good bacteria that reside in the intestines. This provides an opportunity for C. difficile, a bad bacterium, to multiply and take over the intestines without competition from the good bacteria that normally reside in the intestines.

Coronary artery disease – narrowing of the blood vessels that supply oxygen and nutrients to the heart caused by the buildup of fat deposits in the blood vessels and/or hardening of the arteries.

Diuresis – increased urine production. Diuresis is achieved through the use of diuretic drugs (loop diuretics, thiazide diuretics, and potassium-sparing diuretics).

Edema – swelling caused by the presence of excess fluid in the body.

Electrolytes – electrically-charged minerals. Electrolytes, like potassium, calcium, and sodium, are essential for normal body functions (e.g. muscle contraction and nerve function).

Elimination – the excretion of a waste product from the body (e.g via urination).

Embolism – obstruction of a blood vessel by an object; for example, a blood clot or an air bubble.

Emesis – the process of vomiting.

Epistaxis – nosebleed.

Expectorant – an agent used to thin mucus and make it easier to expel/cough up. The most commonly used expectorant for outpatients is the drug guaifenesin (Mucinex®, Robitussin®). For inpatients, inhaled acetylcysteine (Mucomyst®) is probably the most commonly used expectorant. Another term for "expectorant" is "mucolytic agent."

Glaucoma – a disease of the eye characterzed by increased pressure within the eye.

Gout – uric acid levels get too high in the bloodstream and uric acid crystals form. The uric acid crystals (also referred to as "urate crystals") deposit in the joints. The body's immune system attacks the uric acid crystal as a foreign invader, resulting in a big red, inflamed, painful joint.

Heart failure – a condition in which the heart is unable to work hard/effectively enough to meet the body's oxygen needs. Remember that blood functions to carry oxygen to all areas of the body, and the heart is solely responsible for providing the force necessary to circulate the blood through the body.

High efficiency particulate air (HEPA) filter – an air filter that removes 99.97% of particles that are 0.3 microns (0.00003 centimeters) or larger.

Hyperglycemia – abnormally high blood glucose levels.

Hyperkalemia – abnormally high level of potassium in the blood.

Hypertension – high blood pressure.

Hyperuricemia – abnormally high uric acid levels in the blood. Uric acid gets into the bloodstream from dietary intake (certain foods and beverages) and normal cell turnover (many types of cells in the body are dying and being replaced by new cells). Certain drugs can also increase uric acid levels in the blood. This is a problem because when the concentration of uric acid gets too high, the uric acid crystallizes (i.e. turns to a solid), deposits in the joint spaces (usually the joint in the big toe), and causes severe pain and inflammation (i.e. gout).

Hypoglycemia – abnormally low blood glucose levels.

Hypokalemia – low potassium levels in the blood. Potassium is essential for normal muscle and nerve function. Patients with low potassium levels may exhibit muscle weakness and cardiac arrhythmias. Hypokalemia can be caused by thiazide and loop diuretics.

Hypotension – low blood pressure.

Indication – a condition, disease, or disorder for which a drug has been found to be effective in treating. For example, lisinopril is indicated for the treatment of hypertension. In other words, lisinopril has been found to be effective at lowering high blood pressure.

ISO classification – the rating of the quality of the air in a clean room. ISO stands for the International Organization for Standardization. The ISO defines ISO class 8 air as having 3,520,000 particles or less (of size 0.5 microns or larger) per cubic meter, ISO class 7 air as having 352,000 particles or less (of size 0.5 microns or larger) per cubic meter, and ISO class 5 air as having 3,520 particles or less (of size 0.5 microns or larger) per cubic meter. When compounding sterile products for infusion, it is important to use an environment with the very few particles. If a foreign particle gets into the compounded sterile product, it could be infused into the patient's bloodstream and get clogged in a blood vessel. Particles can also be microorganisms (e.g. bacteria, fungi, viruses). The last thing you want to do is infuse microorganisms into a sick patient's vein. Why does sterile compounding usually take place within a hood or workbench located within a clean room? Because clean rooms contain filtered air with a low particle count and hoods/workbenches (e.g. laminar airflow hoods) take that low particle air from the clean room and filter it even more to create a flow of ultra-low particle air directly over the workbench where the compounding takes place.

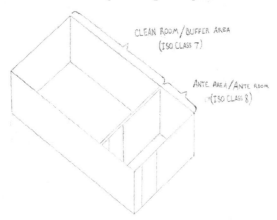

CLEAN ROOM / BUFFER AREA
(ISO CLASS 7)

ANTE AREA / ANTE ROOM
(ISO CLASS 8)

Lacrimation – the production of tears.

Laminar airflow hood (LAFH) – a combined air filtration machine and workbench. The LAFH collects air from its direct surrounding environment, usually a clean room, passes it through two filters (a standard filter and a HEPA filter), and then pushes the filtered air accross the workbench to create an ultra-low particle environment that is ideal for compounding sterile products.

Metabolism – the body's natural process of chemically altering or breaking down a substance (e.g. a drug) to the end of removing the substance from the body.

Myocardial infarction (MI) – an event in which a portion of the heart muscle tissue dies due to a blockage of the coronary artery by a blood clot or a clump of fat (referred to as a "fatty plaque") that breaks off of the wall of a blood vessel and lodges in the coronary artery (see the illustration on the below).

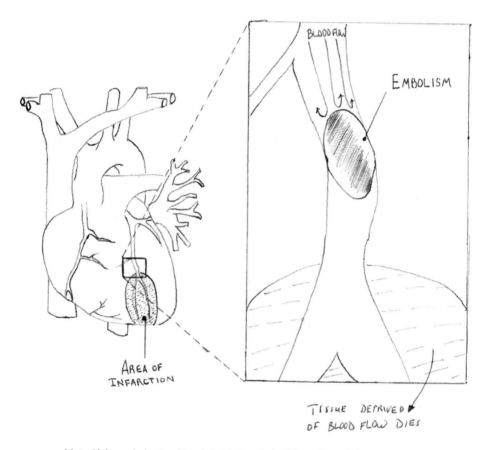

Note: If the embolus is a blood clot, it is called a "thromboembolism."

Nephron – the basic unit of the kidney. Diuretic drugs work by modulating electrolyte exchange at certain locations in the nephron; for example, loop diuretics prevent sodium from being re-absorbed from the Loop of Henle (a segment of the nephron).

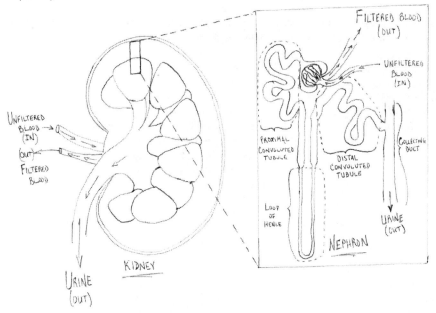

Neuron – a nerve cell; the most basic unit of the nervous system.

Neurotransmitter – a chemical produced within the body that modifies the nervous system.

Nonproductive cough – a dry cough (little-to-no mucous is involved).

Peripheral Neuropathy – tingling and pain in the extremities (fingers and/or toes) resulting from nerve damage. Peripheral neuropathy is most commonly seen in patients with poorly-managed diabetes; the chronically high concentration of glucose in the blood has a damaging effect on nerve cells.

Photosensitivity – increased sensitiy to sunlight which results in a predisposition to sunburn.

Polyuria – excessive production of urine.

Pregnancy category – the FDA created 5 categories to identify the birth defect risk of using a drug during pregnancy. The pregnancy categories are "A, B, C, D, and X." Drugs in pregnancy category A are considered to be the least likely to cause birth defects. Drugs in pregnancy category X are considered to be the most likely to cause birth defects if used during pregnancy. Drugs in pregnancy category X should never be used by someone who is pregnant. The use of a drug in pregnancy category A, B, C, or D may be appropriate if the benefits outweigh the risks.

Priapism – a painful, prolonged erection.

QT interval – the time between the Q wave and T wave on an electrocardiogram. An electrocardiogram is a graph that depicts the flow of electrical impulses through the heart. The electrical impulses cause contraction and relaxation of cardiac (heart) muscle tissue. The reason we are looking at QT interval is that certain drugs can prolong the QT interval, and a prolonged QT interval is a risk factor for life-threatening cardiac arrhythmias that could result in sudden death.

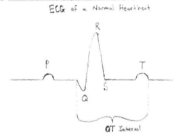

Renal – pertaining to the kidney (e.g. renal failure and kidney failure are synonymous). The kidneys function as a filtration system for blood.

Serotonin syndrome – a condition characterized by mental status changes (e.g. agitation, confusion, hallucinations), pressured speech, tremor, rigidity, diarrhea, fever, sweating, flushing, and/or seizures. Serotonin syndrome is caused by excessive stimulation of serotonin receptors (i.e. taking too many drugs that increase serotonin activity). For example, serotonin syndrome may occur in a patient that takes a combination of fluoxetine, bupropion, and sumatriptan.

Side effects – the undesired consequenses of medication use.

Stevens-Johnson syndrome (SJS) – a disease characterized by fever and a severe skin rash involving the mouth, eyes, and vaginal mucous membranes. The rash causes widespread skin loss which can lead to dehydration, infection, and even death. Toxic Epidermal Necrolysis (TEN) is thought to be a variant of the same condition. Stevens Johnson Syndrome and Toxic Epidermal Necrolysis are usually caused by drugs. There are about 200 drugs that are associated with SJS/TEN, most commonly sulfa antibiotics (e.g. sulfamethoxazole, sulfadiazine) and anticonvulsants (e.g. lamotrigine, phenytoin, valproic acid, carbemazepine, ethosuximide). It should be noted, however, that SJS and TEN are very rare; about 1 in 1,000,000 people per year experience SJS.

Stroke – an event in which a portion of nerve tissue in the brain dies due to interruption of blood flow to the brain.

Sulfa allergy – an allergy to the chemical structure of $-SO_2NH_2$ which is predominantly seen in a class of antibiotics called sulfonamides (e.g. sulfamethoxazole, which is one of the two active ingredients found in the medication known as Bactrim® or Septra®). Certain diuretics, NSAIDs, and anti-diabetic drugs also contain – SO_2NH_2 as part of their chemical structure; therefore, these drugs can trigger an allergic reaction in patients with a sulfa allergy. Many patients with a sulfa allergy mistakenly believe that they are allergic to sulfur or sulfites. Sulfur is found in matchheads, fertilizers, and many other common products, and sulfites are found in common food products as preservatives. However, "sulfa allergy" is an allergy to a particular chemical component found in certain drugs and is *not* the same thing as a "sulfur allergy" or a "sulfite allergy."

Symptom – a sign that indicates the presence of a condition, disease, or disorder. For example, a sore throat, nasal congestion, mild fever, sneezing and cough are signs that inidicate the presence of the common cold.

Syncope – passing out/fainting.

Tachycardia – above normal heart rate at rest. (Normal resting heart rate is 60-90 beats per minute.)

Tolerance – decreased sensitivity to a drug and the capacity to endure large doses with minimal adverse effects.

Veins – the blood vessels that carry blood from the organs back to the heart.

Withdrawal – the response to discontinuing a drug to which a person has become physically or psychologically dependent.

Now that we have reviewed important terms and concepts, we are ready to move on to the specific topics outlined on the PTCB exam blueprint. We'll try to fill in other gaps in knowledge you may have as we go along. So, let's start with Knowledge Domain #1 from the PTCB exam blueprint – "Pharmacology for Technicians."

KNOWLEDGE DOMAIN #1
PHARMACOLOGY FOR TECHNICIANS
(13.75% OF EXAM)

Drugs are grouped into categories – referred to as "drug classes" – based on their pharmacology. Drugs within the same drug class share the same "mechanism of action." Studying the pharmacology of one drug at a time is a tedious and inefficient approach. To simplify and expedite the process, we are going to study pharmacology one drug class at a time. We will be covering uses (indications), mechanisms of action (MoA), side effects (SE), and common drug interactions (DI).

For this section you should study all of the information provided, but make an extra special effort to memorize the drug names and highlighted details. For instance, the first drug class we will review is the ACE inhibitors. Review all of the information on the following page to gain a basic understanding of ACE inhibitors, but before moving on the next drug class (ARBs), make sure you know that Prinivil® (lisinopril), Zestril® (lisinopril), Vasotec® (enalapril), Lotensin® (benazepril), Accupril® (quinapril), and Altace® (ramipril) are all ACE inhibitors that can be used to treat hypertension (high blood pressure). Also know that ACE inhibitors may cause hypotension (low blood pressure) and/or dry cough, may interact with potassium supplements, and should never be used by pregnant women. These are the major points you will learn by focusing on the drug names and highlighted details.

Brand Name	Generic Name
Prinivil®, Zestril®	Lisinopril
Vasotec®	Enalapril
Lotensin®	Benazepril
Accupril®	Quinapril
Altace®	Ramipril

Note: notice how the generic names of the ACE inhibitors end in "-pril."

Indications: Hypertension, Heart Failure, Myocardial Infarction (Heart Attack), Renal Protection in Diabetes Mellitus

MoA: Inhibits angiotensin converting enzyme (ACE), thus preventing the conversion of angiotensin I to angiotensin II. Angiotensin II is a potent vasoconstrictor; constricts blood vessels leading to an increase in blood pressure. Angiotensin II also stimulates secretion of aldosterone, a mineralocorticoid secreted by the kidneys. Aldosterone increases sodium levels in the blood. Since water follows sodium via osmosis, aldosterone secretion ultimately leads to an increase in blood volume and an increase in blood pressure. ACE inhibitors prevent this from taking place.

SE: Dry cough, hypotension, hyperkalemia, anaphylaxis (rare)

DI: Potassium supplements used together with ACE inhibitors may lead to dangerously high potassium levels in the blood which can cause life-threatening cardiac arrhythmias.

Notes: ACE inhibitors cause fetal toxicity and should not be used by pregnant women (pregnancy category X). About 20% of patients on ACE inhibitors experience a dry, nonproductive cough. The only way to eliminate this side effect is to discontinue the ACE inhibitor. Switch to an ARB for the same pharmacologic effect without the dry cough side effect.

Brand Name	Generic Name
Cozaar®	Losartan
Avapro®	Irbesartan
Diovan®	Valsartan
Benicar®	Olmesartan
Micardis®	Telmisartan
Atacand®	Candesartan
Edarbi®	Azilsartan

Note: notice how the generic names of the ARBs end "–sartan."

Indications: Hypertension, Heart Failure, Myocardial Infarction (Heart Attack) Stroke Prevention, Renal Protection in Diabetes Mellitus

MoA: Antagonizes angiotensin II at type 1 angiotensin II receptors (AT1 receptors) found on the blood vessels and heart. The antagonism of angiotensin II leads to relaxation of vascular smooth muscle.

SE: Fatigue, dizziness, hyperkalemia, hypotension, angioedema (rare), anaphylaxis (rare). Since the ARBs do not interfere with bradykinin metabolism, they are not associated with the dry cough side effect seen with ACE inhibitor use.

DI: Since ARBs can increase potassium levels, potassium supplements and potassium-containing salt substitutes can increase the risk of hyperkalemia.

Notes: ARBs cause fetal/neonatal toxicity and should not be used by pregnant women (pregnancy category X).

Brand Name	Generic Name
Microzide®	Hydrochlorothiazide
Diuril®	Chlorthiazide
Zaroxolyn®	Metolzaone
Hygroton®, Thalitone®	Chlorthalidone
Lozol®	Indapamide

Indications: Hypertension, Peripheral Edema

MoA: Decreases NaCl reabsorption at the distal convoluted tubule (DTC) of the nephron by inhibiting the Na+–Cl- symporter. As a result, more sodium remains in the urine. Water follows sodium via osmosis, so the volume of urine output increases (and blood volume decreases).

SE: Hyperglycemia, hyperuricemia, hypokalemia, muscle cramps (related to electrolyte imbalances), cardiac arrhythmias (also related to electrolyte imbalances), photosensitivity (predisposition to sunburn), Stevens-Johnson syndrome (SJS; rare)

DI: Additive hypotension when combined with other drugs that can cause hypotension; additive hypokalemia when administered with loop diuretics; opposes uric acid lowering drugs like allopurinol; can increase blood sugar (monitor blood sugar closely in diabetic patients that are beginning or discontinuing the use of a thiazide diuretic).

Notes: Thiazides contain a sulfonamide component, which may elicit an allergic reaction in patients with a sulfa allergy. Unlike loop diuretics, thiazides have a ceiling effect on diuresis and can only increase urine output up to a certain extent. Judging from the image on the following page, one might venture a guess that diuretics cause hyperkalemia; however, further downstream in the nephron a lot of the excess sodium in the urine is exchanged for potassium. As a result of this exchange the body loses a lot of potassium, so hypokalemia is associated with the use of thiazide diuretics.

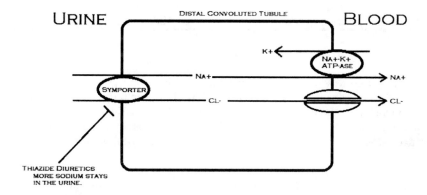

URINE   DISTAL CONVOLUTED TUBULE   BLOOD

THIAZIDE DIURETICS
MORE SODIUM STAYS
IN THE URINE.

****

Drug Interaction –
The "Triple Whammy"

The "Triple Whammy" is the term for the drug interaction between three medications – an NSAID, an ACE or ARB, and a diuretic. When used together, these three medications can cause acute renal damage. NSAIDs inhibit production of prostaglandins, chemicals that work to keep blood vessels feeding the kidneys dilated. ACEs and ARBs cause vasodilation of the efferent arteriole, reducing glomerular filtration pressure. Diuretics cause a reduction in blood flow to the kidneys by reducing blood volume. In other words, all three of these drugs work in different ways that ultimately reduces blood flow to the kidneys. When blood supply is diminished, the cells starve and the organ fails.

****

Brand Name	Generic Name
Bumex®	Bumetanide
Demadex®	Torsemide
Lasix®	Furosemide
Edecrin®	Ethacrynic Acid

Indications: Hypertension, Edema

MoA: Loop diuretics work by blocking the Na-K-Cl$_2$ symporter (a protein that functions to transport sodium, potassium, and chloride ions in a 1:1:2 ratio from the urine to the blood) in the thick ascending limb of the Loop of Henle (a segment of the nephron). Since water follows sodium, this results in increased urinary output which decreases blood volume, and as a result, decreases blood pressure and edema.

SE: Virtually the same side effects as seen with the thiazide diuretics – hyperglycemia, hyperuricemia, hypokalemia, muscle cramps (related to electrolyte imbalances), cardiac arrhythmias (also related to electrolyte imbalances), photosensitivity (predisposition to sunburn), SJS (rare)

DI: Virtually the same drug interactions as seen with the thiazide diuretics – additive hypotension when combined with other drugs that can cause hypotension; additive hypokalemia when administered with loop diuretics; works against drugs that lower uric acid levels (e.g. allopurinol); can increase blood sugar (monitor blood sugar more closely in diabetics starting or stopping thiazides).

Notes: Loop diuretics are the most effective diuretics available. Unlike the thiazides, loop diuretics have no ceiling effect on diuresis. Loop diuretics have the potential to cause life-threatening fluid and electrolyte depletion if used improperly.

****

Pneumonic for Loop Diuretics:

"Beau-Ti-Ful"

When you break the word "beautiful" down into its three syllables (beau-ti-ful), you see that each syllable begins with a letter corresponding to the first letter of the generic name of the most commonly used loop diuretics.

The "B" in Beau- corresponds to the "B" in Bumetanide.
The "T" in -Ti- corresponds to the "T" in Torsemide.
The "F" in –Ful corresponds to the "F" in Furosemide.
****

Brand Name	Generic Name
Dyrenium®	Triamterene
Midamor®	Amiloride
Inspra®	Eplerenone
Aldactone®	Spironolactone

Indications: Hypertension, Heart Failure, Lithium-Induced Polyuria

MoA: Triamterene and Amiloride block sodium-potassium exchange, leading to increased urinary sodium and decreased urinary potassium. Eplerenone and Spironolactone are steroidal compounds that work by antagonizing aldosterone receptors. Aldosterone is a potent mineralocorticoid (causes sodium and water retention).

SE: Spironolactone has some hormonal side effects due to its steroidal chemical structure that can cause gynecomastia in males and breast tenderness in females.

DI: Use of potassium supplements and salt substitutes increases the risk of hyperkalemia.

Notes: Drugs from this class are relatively poor diuretics when compared to loops and thiazides. Potassium-sparing diuretics can be used in combination with loops or thiazides to help avoid potassium imbalances since they have the opposite effect on blood potassium levels.

Brand Name	Generic Name
Flomax®	Tamsulosin
Hytrin®	Terazosin
Cardura®	Doxazosin
Minipress®	Prazosin
Uroxatral®	Afluzosin
Rapaflo®	Silodosin

Note: notice how the generic names of the aplha₁-blockers end "–osin."

Indications: Benign Prostatic Hyperplasia (BPH), Hypertension

MoA: Alpha₁ blockers prevent stimulation of alpha₁ receptors. There are three subtypes of alpha₁ receptors: 1A, 1B, and 1D. Stimulation of the alpha₁ₐ receptor subtype causes contraction of smooth muscles in the bladder neck and prostate. Benign prostatic hyperplasia is characterized by an enlarged prostate that obstructs urine outflow at the level of the bladder neck (the prostate gland encompasses the bladder neck). By selectively blocking the alpha₁ₐ receptor subtype, the muscle in the prostate and bladder neck are relaxed, allowing unobstructed urine outflow. Non-selective alpha₁-blockers cause relaxation of smooth muscle tissue that lines the blood vessels all throughout the body, resulting in decreased peripheral vascular resistance and thus decreased blood pressure.

SE: Orthostatic hypotension (blood pressure drops quickly upon changing from the sitting position to standing), dizziness, syncope, priapism

DI: Increased risk of hypotension when used with other blood pressure lowering drugs.

Brand Name	Generic Name
Catapress®, Kapvay®	Clonidine
Intuniv®, Tenex®	Guanfacine
Aldomet®	Methyldopa

Indications: Hypertension, ADHD

MoA: Activates aplha$_2$-adrenergic receptors. These receptors are found on sympathetic nerve terminals (nerves that release norepinephrine). When activated, alpha$_2$ receptors provide negative feedback to the nerve terminal, which results in decreased norepinephrine output. In simplified terms, activation of alpha$_2$-adrenergic receptors by drugs like clonidine, guanfacine, and methyldopa leads to reduced norepinephrine output by the nervous system. Decreased norepinephrine levels lower the blood pressure.

SE: Bradycardia (slow heart rate), rebound hypertension (a condition that occurs when the medication is withdrawn), dry mouth, impotence, fatigue

DI: Increased risk of hypotension when used with other drugs that decrease blood pressure. Also increases risk of bradycardia when used with drugs that decrease heart rate (e.g. diltiazem, verapamil, and beta-blockers).

Brand Name	Generic Name
Lopressor®	Metoprolol tartrate (immediate-release)
Toprol XL®	Metoprolol succinate (extended-release)
Tenormin®	Atenolol
Coreg®	Carvedilol
Inderal®	Propranolol
Betapace®	Sotalol
Sectral®	Acebutalol
Trandate®	Labetalol
Zebeta®	Bisoprolol

Indications: Hypertension, Angina, Atrial Fibrillation, Myocardial Infarction, Migraines

MoA: β-blockers antagonize β-adrenergic receptors, preventing catecholamines (dopamine, norepinephrine, epinephrine) from binding. This results in decreased chronotropy (slower heart rate), decreased inotropy (less forceful heart beats), and vasodilation (expansion of the blood vessels).

SE: Bradycardia, hypotension, dizziness, fatigue, constipation, diarrhea, dry eyes, male impotence

DI: NSAIDs decrease production of renal prostaglandins, leading to an increase in blood pressure. Some β-blockers interfere with the elimination of diazepam, resulting in higher than expected blood concentrations of diazepam (note: atenolol does not interfere with diazepam metabolism).

Notes: β-blockers should be taken with food. This slows the rate of absorption, decreasing the potential for side effects. Also note that β-blockers blunt the sympathetic response to hypoglycemia, which typically includes sweating, palpitations, and tremor. For diabetic patients that are taking a β-blocker, sweating is the only symptom that is exhibited during an episode of hypoglycemia. Severe cases of hypoglycemia may involve seizure or coma. Abrupt cessation of a β-blocker drug may exacerbate angina, potentially leading to myocardial infarction. For this reason, when discontinuing β-blocker therapy, the dose should be decreased gradually over the course of one to two weeks.

Brand Name	Generic Name
Norvasc®	Amlodipine
Procardia®	Nifedipine
Cardene®	Nicardipine
Plendil®	Felodipine
Sular®	Nisoldipine
Cardizem®, Tiazac®, Taztia XT®	Diltiazem
Isoptin®, Verelan®, Calan®	Verapamil

Indications: Hypertension, Angina, Coronary Artery Disease

MoA: Calcium channel blockers work by blocking the flow of calcium ions into cardiac and vascular smooth muscle cells, which rely on calcium for contraction. The effect is relaxation of cardiac and vascular smooth muscle (the blood vessels dilate, thus blood pressure is reduced) and a decrease in cardiac contractility (the heart contracts less forcefully, thus the heart demands less oxygen. Drugs from this drug class can be used to treat angina*.

SE: Fatigue, edema

DI: Patients on amlodipine should not take more than 20 mg of simvastatin daily due to increased risk of rhabdomyolysis; strong inhibitors of CYP3A4 increase plasma concentrations of amlodipine, which could lead to hypotension and an increase in side effects. The risk of hypotension increases when taken with other drugs that lower blood pressure.

*Angina is chest pain resulting from inadequate blood flow to the heart.

Brand Name	Generic Name
Viagra®, Revatio®	Sildenafil
Cialis®	Tadalafil
Levitra®, Staxyn®	Vardenafil

Indications: Erectile Dysfunction, Pulmonary Arterial Hypertension (Revatio® only)

MoA: PDE-5 inhibitors work by blocking the enzyme known as "phosphodiesterase-5." By blocking PDE-5, the effect of nitric oxide is prolonged. Nitric oxide is a potent vasodilator. Vasodilation increases blood flow. Phosphodiesterase-5 is present in pulmonary vascular smooth muscle (i.e. in blood vessels inside the lungs) and the corpus cavernosum (i.e. the tissue that comprises the inside of the penis), thus PDE-5 inhibitors increase blood flow specifically to these two areas of the body.

SE: Hypotension, headache, epistaxis , and priapism

DI: Increased risk of hypotension when used with other medications that can lower blood pressure (especially nitroglycerin); increased risk of epistaxis (nosebleed) when used with anticoagulant or antiplatelet drugs.

CROSS SECTION OF A BLOOD VESSEL

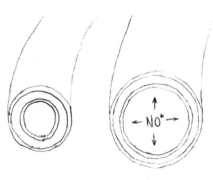

← NO* →

* NO = Nitric Oxide

PDE-5 IS AN ENZYME LOCATED PREDOMINANTLY IN THE BLOOD VESSELS THAT SUPPLY BLOOD TO THE PENIS.

PDE-5 REDUCES THE EFFECT OF NITRIC OXIDE.

BY INHIBITING PDE-5, THE EFFECT OF NITRIC OXIDE IS ENHANCED.

Brand Name	Generic Name
Zocor®	Simvastatin
Lipitor®	Atorvastatin
Crestor®	Rosuvastatin
Pravachol®	Pravastatin
Lescol®	Fluvastatin
Mevacor®	Lovastatin
Livalo®	Pitavastatin

Indications: Hypercholesterolemia (high cholesterol)

MoA: Cholesterol comes from two sources: dietary intake (by eating certain foods) and natural production of cholesterol inside the body. Statins work by inhibiting the enzyme HMG-CoA reductase, which is a key enzyme involved in the normal production of cholesterol. Most cholesterol produced in the human body is produced during the night, so statins are generally more effective when taken at night. Certain statins (e.g. atorvastatin and rosuvastatin) are eliminated from the body at a very slow rate, as these drugs have a long half-life. For this reason, it is not necessary to take atorvastatin or rosuvastatin at night; they can be taken at any time of the day. Since HMG-CoA reductase inhibitors only affect cholesterol production and not dietary intake of cholesterol, patients on a statin should also implement dietary changes to reduce the amount of cholesterol they consume from the foods they eat.

SE: Muscle aches, constipation, liver impairment, myopathy, rhabdomyolysis (rare)

DI: Most drug interactions involving statins increase the risk of myopathy. For drugs in this class, the enzymes responsible for metabolism vary from one statin to the next, but, in general, drugs that inhibit or induce certain CYP450 enzymes (e.g. ketoconazole, cyclosporine, carbamazepine, high quantities of grapefruit juice) lead to decreased or increased metabolism of statins. Enzyme inhibitors decrease the metabolism of the statin, which accumulates in the body. Enzyme inducers increase the metabolism of the statin and ultimately decrease the statin's effectivenes.

Notes: Pregnancy category X.

Brand Name	Generic Name
Pacerone®	Amiodarone
Lanoxin®	Digoxin
Quinalan®	Quinidine
Norpace®	Disopyramide
Xylocaine®	Lidocaine
Rythmol®	Propafenone
Tambocor®	Flecainide
Tikosyn®	Dofetilide

Indications: Cardiac Arrhythmias

MoA: Anti-arrhythmic agents slow down/stabilize the nerve impulses that travel through the heart tissue.

SE: New or worsened arrhythmias, liver damage, visual disturbances, dizziness, fatigue, nausea/vomiting

DI: When taken with drugs that prolong the QT interval (e.g. citalopram, moxifloxacin, tacrolimus, ziprasidone), life-threatening cardiac arrhythmias can result.

Brand Name	Generic Name
AtroPen®	Atropine
Dramamine®	Dimenhydrinate
Antivert®, Bonine®, Dramamine® II	Meclizine
Transderm-Scop®	Scopolamine

Indications: Nausea/Vomiting, Vertigo, Delirium Tremens

MoA: Anticholinergics work by inhibiting the action of acetylcholine (Ach). Acetylcholine is a parasympathetic neurotransmitter. The parasympathetic nervous system is responsible for "rest and digest" activity (e.g. slowing of the heart, contraction of GI smooth muscle, increased digestive gland secretions, constriction of the pupils, and constriction of the bronchioles) whereas the sympathetic nervous system is responsible for "fight or flight" activity (e.g. increased heart rate, dilation of pupils, and dilation of bronchioles). Anticholinergic drugs are also known as "parasympatholytics" ("-lytic" coming from the Greek word "lysis" meaning to break) because they oppose the effects of parasympathetic nervous system.

SE: Cholinergic effects are summarized by the acronym "SLUDGE"

> S – Salivation
> L – Lacrimation
> U – Urination
> D – Defecation
> G – Glandular Secretions
> E – Emesis

Since anticholinergic drugs block, or reduce, cholinergic activity, side effects are predictable (e.g. dry mouth, dry eye, urinary retention, constipation).

DI: Anticholinergics should not be used in patients with narrow angle glaucoma, as these drugs will increase intraocular pressure and worsen the glaucoma. Also, antacids that contain aluminum and/or magnesium may decrease absorption of orally administered anticholinergics.

Brand Name	Generic Name
Prozac®	Fluoxetine
Paxil®	Paroxetine
Zoloft®	Sertraline
Celexa®	Citalopram
Lexapro®	Escitalopram
Luvox®	Fluvoxamine

Indications: Depression, Behavioral Disorders, Eating Disorders

MoA: Serotonin (chemical name: 5-hydroxytryptamine (5-HT)) is a neurotransmitter that plays a key role in depression, behavior, eating, and nausea/vomiting. Serotonin must be available in the the synaptic cleft (the open space between neurons) long enough to exert an effect. When neurons reabsorb (or "reuptake") serotonin, the serotonin is effectively removed from the synaptic cleft and rendered inactive. SSRIs block the reuptake of serotonin, allowing the neurotransmitter to remain in the synaptic cleft where it has more time to exert its effect.

SE: Weight gain or weight loss, reduced sex drive, dry mouth, nausea, diarrhea, serotonin syndrome

****
Symptoms of Serotonin Syndrome
Changes in mental status (e.g. agitation, confusion, hallucinations), pressured speech, tremor*, rigidity, diarrhea, fever, sweating, flushing, and seizures.

*Tremor is the hallmark symptom of serotonin syndrome.
****

DI: Increased risk of bleeding when used with NSAIDs, anticoagulants, and/or antiplatelets; increased risk of serotonin syndrome when used with other medications that increase the effect of serotonin (e.g. SNRIs, triptans, tramadol).

Notes: All antidepressants have the potential to cause suicidal ideation and behavior in patients 24 years of age and younger.

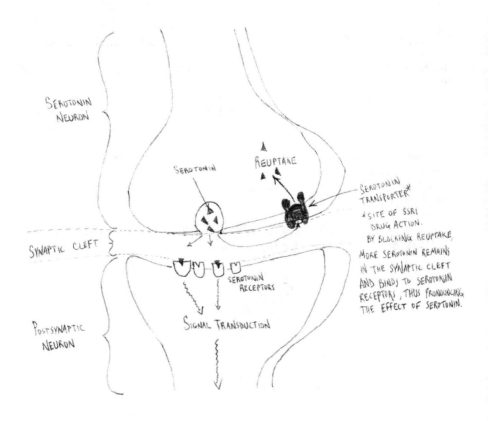

SEROTONIN
NEURON

SEROTONIN

REUPTAKE

SEROTONIN
TRANSPORTER*

*SITE OF SSRI
DRUG ACTION.
BY BLOCKING REUPTAKE,
MORE SEROTONIN REMAINS
IN THE SYNAPTIC CLEFT
AND BINDS TO SEROTONIN
RECEPTORS, THUS PRODUCING
THE EFFECT OF SEROTONIN.

SYNAPTIC CLEFT

SEROTONIN
RECEPTORS

POSTSYNAPTIC
NEURON

SIGNAL TRANSDUCTION

Brand Name	Generic Name
Cymbalta®	Duloxetine
Effexor®	Venlafaxine
Pristiq®	Desvenlafaxine
Savella®	Milnacipran

Indications: Depression, Eating Disorders, Generalized Anxiety Disorder, Diabetic Peripheral Neuropathy

MoA: SNRIs work just like SSRIs, but they also inhibit the reuptake of norepinephrine by adrenergic neurons.

SE: Side effects of SNRIs are similar to those of SSRIs (e.g. serotonin syndrome), but with additional cardiovascular side effects (e.g. heart palpitations, increased blood pressure, tachycardia). Common side effects include dry mouth, nausea, headache, fatigue, and dizziness.

DI: Increased risk of serotonin syndrome when taken with other drugs that increase the activity of serotonin (e.g. SSRIs, triptans, tramadol).

Brand Name	Generic Name
Apidra®	Insulin Glulisine
NovoLog®	Insulin Aspart
Humalog®	Insulin Lispro
Humalog 75/25®	Mixture of 75% Lispro Protamine Insulin and 25% Lispro Insulin
Humulin R®, Novolin R®	Regular Human Insulin
Humulin N®, Novolin N®	Insulin NPH
Novolin 70/30®, Humulin 70/30®	Mixture of 70% Insulin NPH and 30% Regular Human Insulin
Lantus®	Insulin Glargine
Levemir®	Insulin Detemir
Tresiba®	Insulin Degludec

Indications: Type I Diabetes Mellitus, Type II Diabetes Mellitus

MoA: Insulin stimulates cellular uptake of glucose from the blood. There are several different insulin formulations. They are categorized based on how quickly they start working (onset of action) and how long they work (duration of action).

Category	Brand Name	Onset of Action	Duration of Action
Rapid Acting	Apidra®, Humalog®, NovoLog®	15 - 30 min.	3 - 6 hours
Short Acting	Humulin R®, Novolin R®	30 - 60 min.	6 - 10 hours
Intermediate Acting	Humulin N®, Novolin N®	1 - 2 hours	16 - 24 hours
Long Acting	Lantus®, Levemir®	1 - 2 hours	24 hours
Ultra Long Acting	Tresiba®	1 hour	24 - 40 hours

SE: Hypoglycemia, redness/swelling/itching at injection site

DI: Several drugs (e.g. thyroid hormones, diuretics, corticosteroids) can increase blood sugar, opposing the effect of insulin. Likewise, several drugs (e.g. oral antidiabetics, fibrates) can decrease blood sugar and have additive blood sugar lowering effects.

Notes: **KEEP REFRIGERATED** until dispensed. Insulin expires 28 days after the rubber stopper of the vial is punctured with a needle. With the exception of U-500 insulin, the concentration of all insulin is 100 units per milliliter (each 0.01 mL of liquid contains 1 unit of insulin). With U-500 insulin, the concentration is 500 units per milliliter (each 0.01 mL of liquid contains 5 unit of insulin).

Insulin Formulations Available Without a Prescription (OTC)

Novolin N	Novolin R	Novolin 70/30
Humulin N	Humulin R	Humulin 70/30

****

A Word On Diabetes

Cells need glucose in order to survive. Insulin gives cells the ability to access glucose present in the blood. Patients with type I diabetes do not produce enough insulin to survive; therefore, these patients require insulin. Patients with type II diabetes do not always require therapy with insulin. Many type II diabetes patients can control their blood sugar levels with diet, exercise, and oral antidiabetics (e.g. sulfonylureas, DPP-4 inhibitors, and metformin).

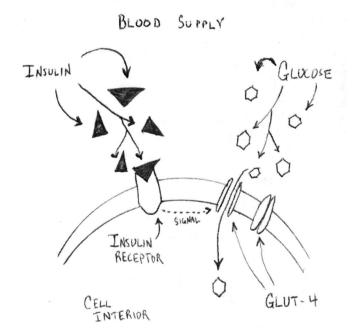

Brand Name	Generic Name
Glucophage®, Fortamet®	Metformin

Indications: Type II Diabetes Mellitus

MoA: Lowers blood glucose by three mechanisms:
1. Decreases amount of glucose produced by the liver.
2. Decreases intestinal absorption of glucose.
3. Improves cellular response to insulin.

Note: Metformin does not work by increasing insulin secretion; therefore, it does not have the potential to cause hypoglycemia as some other oral antidiabetics do.

SE: Lactic acidosis, vitamin B12 deficiency, diarrhea, nausea/vomiting

DI: Cimetidine can increase metformin levels by up to 50%.

Brand Name	Generic Name
Januvia®	Sitagliptin
Onglyza®	Saxagliptin
Tradjenta®	Linagliptin
Nesina®	Alogliptin

Indications: Type II Diabetes Mellitus

MoA: DPP-4 inhibitors lower blood glucose by preventing the degradation of incretins. Naturally present in the human body, incretins increase insulin secretion and decrease glucagon secretion. By preserving incretins, more glucose is absorbed by cells via insulin, and less glucose is mobilized into the bloodstream by glucagon.

SE: Hypoglycemia (low-risk), musculoskeletal pain, headache, upper respiratory infection, Stevens-Johnson syndrome (SJS; rare)

DI: Increased risk of hypoglycemia when used in combination with sulfonylureas (especially glyburide) and/or insulin. CYP3A4 inducers (e.g. rifampin) can reduce the effect of saxagliptin and linagliptin. CYP3A4 inhibitors (e.g. ketoconazole, clarithromycin) can increase the effect of saxagliptin and linagliptin.

Brand Name	Generic Name
Amaryl®	Glimepiride
Glucotrol®	Glipizide
DiaBeta®, Micronase®	Glyburide
Tolinase®	Tolazamide
Tol-tab®	Tolbutamide
Diabinese®	Chlorpropamide

Indications: Type II Diabetes Mellitus

MoA: Cells obtain the fuel they need to survive from glucose in the blood. Insulin allows cells to take up glucose from the blood. In type II diabetes, it is theorized that one of three things is taking place – 1) the cells are not responsive to insulin, 2) not enough insulin is being secreted from the pancreas, or 3) both 1 & 2 are occurring at the same time. Since the glucose is not being used by the cells, it builds up in the blood. This high concentration of glucose in the blood damages blood vessels and nerve cells. Severe damage to the blood vessels in the kidneys (leading to renal failure) and the nerves of the eye (leading to blindness) are typical of consequences of untreated, or poorly managed, diabetes. Sulfonylureas are known as "secretagogues," which means they work by stimulating insulin secretion.

SE: Since sulfonylureas stimulate insulin secretion, hypoglycemia is a side effect (more severe with glyburide; especially when dietary intake is limited). Another common side effect is weight gain (also more severe with glyburide).

DI: Many drugs (e.g. quinolones, anticoagulants, azole antifungals, MAOIs) can increase the hypoglycemic effect of sulfonylureas. Likewise, many drugs (e.g. thyroid hormones, diuretics, corticosteroids, beta-blockers, calcium channel blockers) can reduce the effect of sulfonylureas. Also worth noting, alcohol can prolong the effect of glipizide and cause a disulfiram-like reaction in patients taking chlorpropamide.

Notes: Use of 2nd generation sulfonylureas (glimepiride, glipizide, glyburide) is preferred over 1st generation sulfonylureas (tolazamide, tolbutamide, chlorpropamide).

Brand Name	Generic Name
Prilosec®	Omeprazole
Nexium®	Esomeprazole
Protonix®	Pantoprazole
Prevacid®	Lansoprazole
AciPhex®	Rabeprazole

Indications: Gastroesophageal Reflux Disease (GERD), Peptic Ulcer Disease (PUD), Barrett's Esophagus

MoA: An enzyme known as Hydrogen-Potassium ATPase, or the "proton pump," is responsible for secreting acid (i.e. hydrogen ions) into the stomach by exchanging potassium ions from the stomach for hydrogen ions (i.e. acid). Proton pump inhibitors block this enzyme (Hydrogen-Potassium ATPase) and prevent it from functioning. This greatly reduces the amount of acid in the stomach.

SE: Abdominal pain, headache, diarrhea, nausea/vomiting, clostridium difficile diarrhea, bone fractures

DI: The most well-known drug interaction involving PPIs is probably the one between omeprazole and clopidogrel. Clopidogrel must be activated by the enzyme CYP2C19 in order to be effective. Omeprazole (and esomeprazole – an isomer of omeprazole) inhibits CYP2C19. As a result, the effect of clopidogrel is reduced when used in conjunction with omeprazole or esomeprazole. Also, some drugs (e.g. levothyroxine) rely on stomach acid for optimal absorption. Since PPIs reduce stomach acid, absorption of some other drugs may be impaired.

Notes: In patients with clostridium difficile diarrhea (pseudomembranous colitis), use of proton pump inhibitors increases the probability that the clostridium difficile infection will recur.

Brand Name	Generic Name
Zantac®	Ranitidine
Pepcid®	Famotidine
Tagamet®	Cimetidine
Axid®	Nizatidine

Indications: Gastroesophageal Reflux Disease (GERD), Peptic Ulcer Disease (PUD)

MoA: Histamine binds to receptors in the stomach that trigger acid release from parietal cells. Histamine-2 (H2) blockers prevent histamine from binding to these receptors, thus reducing acid production in the stomach.

SE: Constipation, headache, seizures (rare), gynecomastia (with cimetidine only)

DI: Some drugs (e.g. levothyroxine) rely on stomach acid for optimal absorption. Since H2 blockers reduce stomach acid, absorption of other drugs can be impaired.

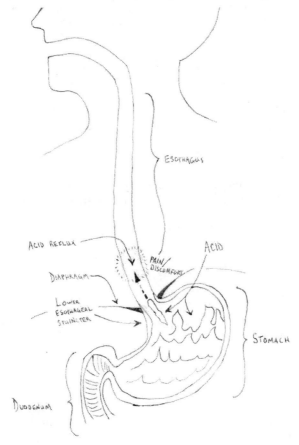

Brand Name	Generic Name
Tegretol®, Epitol®	Carbamazepine
Trileptal®	Oxcarbazepine
Topamax®	Topiramate
Dilantin®	Phenytoin
Neurontin®	Gabapentin
Keppra®	Levetiracetam
Lyrica®	Pregabalin
Vimpat®	Lincosamide
Depakote®	Divalproex
Lamictal®	Lamotrigine
Zonegran®	Zonisamide

Indications: Epilepsy/Seizures, Nerve Pain, Psychiatric Disorders

MoA: Anti-epileptic drugs work by suppressing nerve activity. There are various mechanisms by which this can be accomplished (e.g. sodium ion channel modulation, GABA* receptor stimulation, glutamate** receptor antagonism, benzodiazepine receptor stimulation).

SE: Drowsiness, mental slowing, skin rash, weight gain, liver toxicity, Stevens-Johnson syndrome (rare), increased risk of suicidal thoughts and behavior

DI: Nervous system suppression is greater when combined with other drugs that suppress the nervous system (e.g. benzodiazepines, opioids, alcohol).

*GABA (gamma-aminobutyric acid) is the primary *inhibitory* neurotransmitter of the central nervous system.
** Glutamate is the primary *excitatory* neurotransmitter of the central nervous system. Anti-epileptic drugs are also referred to as anticonvulsants.

Brand Name	Generic Name
Veetids®	Penicillin
Amoxil®	Amoxicillin
Augmentin®	Amoxicillin/Clavulanate
Keflex®	Cephalexin
Cipro®	Ciprofloxacin
Avelox®	Moxifloxacin
Levaquin®	Levofloxacin
Flagyl®	Metronidazole
Zithromax®, Z-pak®	Azithromycin
Biaxin®	Clarithromycin
Vancocin®	Vancomycin
Zosyn®	Piperacillin/Tazobactam
Unasyn®	Ampicillin/Sulbactam

Indications: Bacterial Infections

MoA: There are several different antibiotics with several different mechanisms of action. On a basic level, they all work by exploiting differences between bacterial cells and human cells. For instance, clarithromycin (a macrolide antibiotic) works by binding to the 50S ribosomal subunit of bacterial ribosomes, resulting in inhibition of protein synthesis. Ultimately this kills the cell. Human cells remain unharmed because they do not possess 50S ribosomal subunits.

SE: Diarrhea

DI: Antibiotics increase the effect of warfarin, leading to an increased risk of bleeding in patients taking warfarin. Antibiotics also decrease the effect of oral contraceptives. Oral administration of certain antibiotics should be separated by at least 2 – 4 hours from oral administration of antacids or multivitamins that contain divalent or trivalent cations such as Calcium (Ca^{2+}), Magnesium (Mg^{2+}), Iron (Fe^{2+}/Fe^{3+}), and Aluminum (Al^{3+}).

Notes: Unless directed otherwise by their healthcare provider, a patient should not discontinue antibiotic therapy until the entire prescribed course of treatment has been completed. When antibiotics are discontinued early, the bacteria causing the infection can develop resistance to the antibiotic. By finishing the full course of treatment, the patient is improving the probability that all of the infection-causing bacteria will be eliminated.

Brand Name	Generic Name
Ecotrin®	Aspirin
Motrin®, Advil®	Ibuprofen
Aleve®, Naprosyn®	Naproxen
Mobic®	Meloxicam
Indocin®	Indomethacin
Voltaren®	Diclofenac
Celebrex®	Celecoxib

Indications: Pain, Fever, Rheumatoid Arthritis, Osteoarthritis

MoA: Cyclooxygenase (COX) is an enzyme involved in the creation of prostaglandins and thromboxane. Prostaglandins are chemical mediators of inflammation (i.e. they promote inflammation). Prostaglandins also play a role in protecting the gastric mucosa (the lining of the stomach) from acid-related damage. NSAIDs work by inhibiting COX. There are two subtypes of the cyclooxygenase enzyme: COX-1 and COX-2. Cyclooxygenase-1 is associated with normal physiologic functions (e.g. gastric mucosal protection and blood clotting) and COX-2 is associated with inflammation. Most NSAIDs are non-selective inhibitors of COX (i.e. they inhibit both subtypes, COX-1 and COX-2). Celecoxib is unique because it selectively inhibits COX-2. This is important since inhibition of COX-1 is associated with a higher incidence of gastric mucosal damage. As a result, celecoxib is less irritating to the stomach and less likely than the other NSAIDs to cause or aggravate ulcers of the gastric mucosa. Another unique drug is aspirin. Aspirin is an *irreversible* inhibitor of COX, whereas the other NSAIDs are reversible inhibitors. This irreversible inhibition leads to a more pronounced antiplatelet effect (i.e. prevents blood clot formation), thus aspirin can also be used for heart attack and stroke prevention.

SE: Nausea, vomiting, renal impairment, GI ulceration, hypernatremia and heart failure (increased sodium retention causes increased water retention)

DI: Increased risk of bleeding (especially gastrointestinal bleeding) when used with other drugs that inhibit blood clot formation (i.e. anticoagulants and antiplatelets such as warfarin, clopidogrel, dabigatran, and heparin); increased risk of renal failure when used with other drugs that can impair renal function, such as ACE inhibitors, ARBs, and diuretics.

Brand Name	Generic Name
Roxicodone®	Oxycodone (immediate-release)
Oxycontin®	Oxycodone (extended-release)
Roxanol®	Morphine (immediate-release)
MS Contin®, Kadian®	Morphine (extended-release)
Dilaudid®	Hydromorphone
various combination products*	Codeine
various combination products**	Hydrocodone

* Robitussin® AC, Tylenol® #3, etc.
** Norco®, Lortab®, Vicodin®, Tussionex®, Tussigon®, etc.

Indications: Pain, Cough

MoA: Agonist at opioid receptors, particularly mu (μ) opioid receptors. Mu (μ) opioid receptors are involved in pain and wakefulness; thus, pain relief and sedation are associated with opioid drug use.

SE: Sedation, respiratory depression, constipation

DI: Increased incidence of sedation and respiratory depression when taken with other drugs that suppress the nervous system (e.g. benzodiazepines, alcohol).

Notes: For patients that have used an opioid on a long-term basis, the opioid must be discontinued gradually over time to avoid the symptoms associated with abrupt withdrawal. In general, it is recommended that the dose be decreased by 25-50% per day until discontinued. The patient should be monitored closely during discontinuation. If withdrawal symptoms appear, return to the previous dose and decrease at a slower rate. Take note that constipation is the only side effect to which patients do not develop a tolerance when using opioids.

Opioid Conversion

When converting from one opioid to another, it is safer to underestimate the equivalent dose, as opposed to overestimating. This helps avoid dangerous side effects, like respiratory depression. As a rule of thumb, begin with one-half of the estimated equivalent dose and provide the patient with a rescue supply of additional medication to use for uncontrolled pain.

Brand Name	Generic Name
Ativan®	Lorazepam
Klonopin®	Clonazepam
Halcion®	Triazolam
Versed®	Midazolam
Onfi®	Clobazam
Restoril®	Temazepam
Prosom®	Estazolam
Xanax®	Alprazolam
Valium®, Diastat®	Diazepam
Librium®	Chlordiazepoxide
Tranxene®	Clorazepate

Indications: Insomnia, Anxiety, Agitation, Seizures, Muscle Spasms, Alcohol Withdrawal

MoA: Benzodiazepines bind to benzodiazepine receptors (BNZ_1 and BNZ_2) and enhance the effect of GABA (gamma-aminobutyric acid; the primary inhibitory neurotransmitter of the central nervous system). Specifically, BNZ_1 receptor stimulation promotes sleep and BNZ_2 receptor stimulation promotes muscle relaxation and inhibits memory function.

SE: Drowsiness/somnolence, headache, dizziness, confusion, fatigue

DI: Increased central nervous system depression when taken with other drugs that suppress the nervous system (e.g. non-benzodiazepine sedative-hypnotics, opioids, anticonvulsants, alcohol).

Notes: All drugs in this class are Schedule IV controlled substances according to federal law (individual state laws may be more stringent).

Brand Name	Generic Name
Ambien®	Zolpidem
Lunesta®	Eszopiclone
Sonata®	Zaleplon

Indications: Insomnia

MoA: Similar to benzodiazepines, but drugs in this class tend to bind to BNZ_1 receptors (which promote sleep) more than BNZ_2 receptors.

SE: Drowsiness/somnolence, headache, dizziness

DI: Increased central nervous system depression when taken with other drugs that suppress the nervous system (e.g. benzodiazepines, opioids, anticonvulsants, alcohol).

Notes: All drugs in this class are Schedule IV controlled substances.

The top 238 prescription drugs are listed in this section. Included is the brand name of the drug (if applicable), the generic name in parenthesis, the available strengths, and the route of administration. To interpret abbreviations, refer to the *Abbreviation Legend* below. Drugs are grouped by primary indication (e.g. pain, anxiety, cough). **Note:** Focus on knowing brand & generic names of each drug along with their primary indication.

Abbreviation Legend
TAB/CAP – tablet and/or capsule
SC – subcutaneous injection
IV – intravenous injection or infusion
IM – intramuscular injection
ER – extended release
LA – long acting
DR – delayed release
CR – controlled release
C-II – schedule II controlled substance
C-III – schedule III controlled substance
C-IV – schedule IV controlled substance
C-V – schedule V controlled substance

Underactive Thyroid (Hypothyroidism)
Synthroid®, Levoxyl® (levothyroxine)
25, 50, 75, 88, 100, 112, 125, 137, 150, 175, 200, 300 mcg (TAB/CAP)

Low Potassium (Hypokalemia)
K-Dur®, Klor-Con® (potassium chloride)
8, 10, 15, 20 mEq (TAB/CAP)

Weight Loss
Adipex-P® (phentermine) *C-IV*
37.5 mg (TAB/CAP)

Osteoporosis Treatment/Prevention
Actonel® (risedronate)
5, 30, 35, 150 mg (TAB/CAP)

Boniva® (ibandronate)
150 mg (TAB/CAP)
1 mg/mL solution (IV)

Fosamax® (alendronate)
5, 10, 35, 70 mg (TAB/CAP)
70 mg/75mL (oral solution)

Evista® (raloxifene) *also used for prevention of breast cancer*
60 mg (TAB/CAP)

Malaria
Qualaquin® (quinine)
324 mg (TAB/CAP)

Anxiety
Xanax® (alprazolam) *C-IV*
0.25, 0.5, 1, 2 mg (TAB/CAP)
Note: Xanax® XR is an extended-release tablet available in 0.5, 1, 2, and 3 mg strengths.

Ativan® (lorazepam) *C-IV*
0.5, 1, 2 mg (TAB/CAP)
2 mg/mL, 4 mg/mL (IV solution)

Klonopin® (clonazepam) *C-IV*
0.5, 1, 2 mg (TAB/CAP)

Buspar® (buspirone)
5, 10, 15, 30 mg (TAB/CAP)

Insomnia
Rozerem® (ramelteon)
8 mg (TAB/CAP)

Restoril® (temazepam) *C-IV*
7.5, 15, 22.5, 30 mg (TAB/CAP)

Lunesta® (eszopiclone) *C-IV*
1, 2, 3 mg (TAB/CAP)

Ambien® (zolpidem) *C-IV*
5, 10 mg (TAB/CAP)
Note: Ambien® CR is available in 6.25 and 12.5 mg strengths.

Muscle Spasms
Zanaflex® (tizanidine)
2, 4, 6 mg (TAB/CAP)

Flexeril® (cyclobenzaprine)
5, 10 mg (TAB/CAP)

Skelaxin® (metaxalone)
400, 800 mg (TAB/CAP)

Soma® (carisoprodol) *C-IV*
250, 350 mg (TAB/CAP)

Robaxin® (methocarbamol)
500, 750 mg (TAB/CAP)
100 mg/mL (injection solution)

Liorisal® (baclofen)
10, 20 mg (TAB/CAP)
0.5 mg/mL, 2 mg/mL solution (intrathecal)

Pain
Vicodin® (hydrocodone/acetaminophen) *C-II*
5/300 mg (TAB/CAP)
Note: Vicodin® HP is available as a 10/300 mg tablet and Vicodin® ES is available as a 7.5/300 mg tablet.

Norco® (hydrocodone/acetaminophen) *C-II*
5/325, 7.5/325, 10/325 mg (TAB/CAP)

Endocet® (oxycodone/acetaminophen) *C-II*
5/325, 7.5/325, 10/325 mg (TAB/CAP)

Percocet® (oxycodone/acetaminophen) *C-II*
2.5/325, 5/325, 7.5/325, 10/325 mg (TAB/CAP)

Roxicodone® (oxycodone) *C-II*
5, 15, 30 mg (TAB/CAP)

Oxycontin® (oxycodone ER) *C-II*
10(ER), 15(ER), 20(ER), 30(ER), 40(ER), 60(ER), 80(ER) mg (TAB/CAP)

MS Contin® (morphine) *C-II*
15(ER), 30(ER), 60(ER), 100(ER), 200(ER) mg (TAB/CAP)

Codeine *C-II* *Also a cough suppressant*
15, 30, 60 mg (TAB/CAP)
30 mg/5mL (oral solution)

Methadone *C-II*
5, 10, 40 mg (TAB/CAP)
1, 2, 10 mg/mL (oral solution)
10 mg/mL (injection solution)

Duragesic® (fentanyl) *C-II*
12, 25, 50, 75, 100 mcg/hour (transdermal patch)

Demerol® (meperidine) *C-II*
50, 100 mg (TAB/CAP)
50 mg/mL, 100 mg/mL (injection solution)

Dilaudid® (hydromorphone) *C-II*
2, 4, 8 mg (TAB/CAP)
1 mg/mL (oral solution)
1, 2, 4 mg/mL (injection solution)

Ultram® (tramadol) *C-IV*
50, 100(ER), 200(ER), 300(ER) mg (TAB/CAP)

Ultracet® (tramadol/acetaminophen) *C-IV*
37.5/325 mg (TAB/CAP)

Xilocaine® (lidocaine)
0.5, 1, 2% (injection solution)
2% (mucous membrane solution)
2% (topical jelly)
4% (topical solution)

Lidoderm® (lidocaine)
5% (ER) (topical patch)

Tylenol® #3 (acetaminophen/codeine) *C-III*
30/300 mg (TAB/CAP)

Migraines
Fioricet® (butalbital/acetaminophen/caffeine)
325/50/40 mg (TAB/CAP)

Imitrex® (sumatriptan)
25, 50, 100 mg (TAB/CAP)
6 mg/0.5 mL (SC solution)
5, 20 mg (nasal spray)

Cough
Tussionex® (hydrocodone/chlorpheniramine) *C-II*
8/10 mg/5mL (ER) (oral suspension)

Hycodan®, Hydromet® (hydrocodone/homatropine) *C-II*
5/1.5 mg (TAB/CAP), 5 – 1.5 mg/5mL (oral syrup)

Tessalon® (benzonatate)
100, 200 mg (TAB/CAP)

Cheratussin® AC (guaifenesin/codeine) *C-V*
100/10 mg/5mL (oral syrup)

Cheratussin® DAC (guaifenesin/codeine/pseudoephedrine) *C-V*
100/10/30 mg/5mL (oral syrup)

Psychiatric Disorders
Seroquel® (quetiapine)
25, 50, 100, 200, 300, 400 mg (TAB/CAP)
Note: Seroquel® XR is an extended release version of quetiapine available in 50, 150, 200, 300, and 400 mg formulations.

Risperdal® (risperidone)
0.25, 0.5, 1, 2, 3, 4 mg (TAB/CAP)
1 mg/mL (oral solution)
Note: Risperdal-M® is an orally disintegrating tablet (ODT) available in 0.5, 1, 2, 3, and 4 mg formulations.

Zyprexa® (olanzapine)
2.5, 5, 7.5, 10, 15, 20 mg (TAB/CAP)
Note: Zyprexa is also available as Zyprexa® Zydis (ODT) and Zyprexa® Relprevv (IM injection).

Geodon® (ziprasidone)
20, 40, 60, 80 mg (TAB/CAP)
Note: also available as an IM injection.

Haldol® (haloperidol)
0.5, 1, 2, 5, 10, 20 mg (TAB/CAP)
Note: Haloperidol is also available in an injectable form.

Lithobid®, Eskalith®, Carbolith® (lithium carbonate)
150, 300, 300(ER), 450(CR), 600 mg (TAB/CAP)

Abilify® (aripiprazole)
2, 5, 10, 15, 20, 30 mg (TAB/CAP)
1 mg/mL (oral solution)
Note: aripiprazole is also available in a 10 and 15 mg ODT formulation called Abilify® Discmelts and an IM injection known as Abilify® Maintena.

Seizure Disorders
Dilantin® (phenytoin)
50 mg (chewable tablets)
30, 100(ER) mg (TAB/CAP)
125 mg/5mL (oral suspension)

Depakote® (divalproex)
125, 250, 500(DR) mg (TAB/CAP)
Note: Depakote® ER is an extended release tablet available in 250 and 500 mg; Depakote® Sprinkles are capsules whose contents can be sprinkled into soft food and are available in 125 mg capsules.

Tegretol® (carbamazepine)
100 mg (chewable tablets)
200 mg (TAB/CAP)
100 mg/5mL (oral suspension)

Keppra® (levetiracetam)
250, 500, 750, 1,000 mg (TAB/CAP)
100 mg/mL (oral solution and IV solution)

Trileptal® (Oxcarbazepine)
150, 300, 600 mg (TAB/CAP)
300 mg/5mL (oral suspension)

Topamax® (topiramate)
15, 25, 50, 100, 200 mg (TAB/CAP)

Lamictal® (lamotrigine)
25, 100, 150, 200 mg (TAB/CAP)
Note: lamotrigine is also available as Lamictal® XR in 25, 50, 100, 200, 250, and 300 extended release tablets.

Neurontin® (gabapentin) *also used for nerve pain*
100, 300, 400, 600, 800 mg (TAB/CAP)
50 mg/mL (oral solution)

Valium® (diazepam) *C-IV* *also used for anxiety and muscle spasms*
2, 5, 10 mg (TAB/CAP)
1 mg/mL, 5 mg/mL (oral solution)

Lyrica® (pregabalin) *C-V* *also used for fibromyalgia/nerve pain*
25, 50, 75, 100, 150, 200, 225, 300 mg (TAB/CAP)
20 mg/mL (oral solution)

Parkinson's Disease
Requip® (ropinirole) *also used to treat restless leg syndrome (RLS)*
0.25, 0.5, 1, 2, 3, 4, 5 mg (TAB/CAP)
Note: Requip® XL exists in 2, 4, 6, 8, and 10 mg extended release tablets.

Alzheimer's Disease
Aricept® (donepezil)
5, 5 (ODT), 10, 10(ODT), 23 mg (TAB/CAP)

Namenda® (memantine)
5, 10 mg (TAB/CAP)
7(ER), 14(ER), 21(ER), 28(ER) mg (TAB/CAP)
2 mg/mL (oral solution)

Birth Control
Ortho Cyclen® (norgestimate/ethinyl estradiol)
0.25 mg norgestimate/35 mcg ethinyl estradiol

Depo-Provera® (medroxyprogesterone)
150 mg/mL, 400 mg/mL (injection suspension)

Menopause Symptoms (Hormone Replacement Therapy)
Premarin® (conjugated estrogens)
0.3, 0.45, 0.625, 0.9, 1.25, 2.5 mg (TAB/CAP)
0.625 mg/gram (vaginal cream)

Estrace® (estradiol)
0.5, 1, 2 mg (TAB/CAP)
0.1 mg/gram (vaginal cream)

Evamist® (estradiol)
1.53 mg/actuation (topical spray)

Vagifem® (estradiol)
10 mcg (vaginal tablet)

Overactive Bladder (Urinary Incontinence)
Detrol® (tolterodine)
1, 2 mg (TAB/CAP)
Note: Detrol® LA is available as a 2 and 4 mg extended release tablet.

Ditropan® (oxybutynin)
5, 5(ER), 10(ER), 15(ER) mg (TAB/CAP)
1 mg/mL (oral syrup)

Vesicare® (solifenacin)
5, 10 mg (TAB/CAP)

Nausea/Vomiting (Emesis)
Zofran® (ondansetron)
4, 4(ODT), 8, 8(ODT), 24 mg (TAB/CAP), 4 mg/5mL (oral solution)
2 mg/mL (injection solution)

Phenergan® (promethazine)
12.5, 25, 50 mg (TAB/CAP and rectal supTab/Capsitories)
25 mg/mL, 50 mg/mL (injection solution)

Compazine® (prochlorperazine)
5, 10 mg (TAB/CAP)

Antivert® (meclizine)
12.5, 25, 50 mg (TAB/CAP)

Arthritis
Trexall® (methotrexate) MTX *also used to treat some cancers*
5, 7.5, 10, 15 mg (TAB/CAP)

Inflammation (Steroids)
Medrol® (methylprednisolone)
2, 4, 8, 16, 32 mg (TAB/CAP)

Deltasone® (prednisone)
1, 2.5, 5, 10, 20, 50 mg (TAB/CAP)
1 mg/mL, 5 mg/mL (oral solution)

Decadron® (dexamethasone)
0.5, 0.75, 1, 1.5, 2, 4, 6 mg (TAB/CAP)
0.5 mg/5mL, 5 mg/5mL oral solution
0.5 mg/5mL (elixir)

Cortizone-10® topical (hydrocortisone)
1% (cream, ointment, lotion, gel)

Kenalog® topical (triamcinolone)
0.025, 0.1, 0.5% (cream, ointment, lotion)

Nasacort® AQ (triamcinolone)
55 mcg/actuation (nasal spray)

Inflammation (Non-Steroidal Anti-Inflammatory Drugs (NSAIDs))
Naprosyn® (naproxen)
250, 375, 500 mg (TAB/CAP)
25 mg/mL (oral suspension)

Motrin®, Advil® (ibuprofen)
100 mg (chewable tablets)
200, 400, 600, 800 mg (TAB/CAP)
100 mg/5mL oral suspension and IV solution)

Lodine® (etodolac)
200, 300, 400, 400(ER), 500, 500(ER), 600(ER) mg (TAB/CAP)

Relafen® (nabumetone)
500, 750 mg (TAB/CAP)

Toradol® (ketorolac)
10 mg (TAB/CAP)
15 mg/mL, 30 mg/mL (injection solution)

Indocin® (indomethacin) *commonly used in treatment of gout flares*
25, 50, 75(ER) mg (TAB/CAP)
25 mg/5mL (oral suspension)
50 mg (rectal suppository)

Celebrex® (celecoxib)
50, 100, 200, 400 mg (TAB/CAP)

Voltaren® (diclofenac)
25, 50, 75, 100(ER) mg (TAB/CAP)
1% (topical gel)
0.1% (ophthalmic solution)

Mobic® (meloxicam)
7.5, 15 mg (TAB/CAP)
7.5 mg/5mL (oral suspension)

Allergies
Benadryl® (diphenhydramine)
25, 50 mg (TAB/CAP), 50 mg/mL (injection solution), 2% (topical gel)
12.5 mg/5mL (oral syrup and oral solution), 12.5 mg (ODT)

Zyrtec® (cetirizine)
5, 10 mg (TAB/CAP and chewable tablets), 1 mg/mL (oral syrup)
0.025% (ophthalmic solution)

Atarax® (hydroxyzine)
10, 25, 50 mg (TAB/CAP)
10 mg/5mL (oral syrup)
25 mg/mL, 50 mg/mL (IM solution)

Allegra® (fexofenadine)
30, 30(ODT), 60, 180 mg (TAB/CAP)
30 mg/5mL (oral suspension)

Flonase® (fluticasone)
50 mcg/actuation (nasal spray)

Claritin® (loratadine)
5 mg (chewable tablets), 5(ODT), 10, 10(ODT) mg (TAB/CAP)
5 mg/5mL (oral syrup and oral solution)

Nasonex® (mometasone)
50 mcg/actuation (nasal spray)

Gastroesophageal Reflux Disease (GERD)

Prilosec® (omeprazole)
10(DR), 20(DR), 40(DR) mg (TAB/CAP)

Nexium® (esomeprazole)
20(DR), 40(DR) mg (TAB/CAP)
2.5, 5, 10, 20, 40 mg/packet (oral packets)
20, 40 mg (powder for IV solution)

Protonix® (pantoprazole)
20, 40 mg (TAB/CAP)
40 mg/packet (oral packets)
40 mg (powder for IV solution)

Prevacid® (lansoprazole)
15(DR), 15(ODT), 30(DR), 30(ODT) mg (TAB/CAP)
3 mg/mL (powder for oral suspension)

Dexilant® (dexlansoprazole)
30(DR), 60(DR) mg (TAB/CAP)

Aciphex® (rabeprazole)
20 mg (TAB/CAP)

Pepcid® (famotidine)
10, 20, 20 (chewable tablets), 40 mg (TAB/CAP)
40 mg/5 mL (powder for oral suspension)
0.4 mg/mL, 10 mg/mL (IV solution)

Zantac® (ranitidine)
75, 150, 300 mg (TAB/CAP)
15 mg/mL (oral syrup)
25 mg/mL (injection solution)

Reglan® (metoclopramide)
5, 10 mg (TAB/CAP)
5, 10 mg (ODT)
5 mg/5mL (oral syrup and oral solution)
5 mg/mL (IV solution)

Diabetes Mellitus
Byetta® (exenatide) **KEEP REFRIGERATED**
250 mcg/mL (subcutaneous solution)

Avandia® (rosiglitazone)
2, 4, 8 mg (TAB/CAP)

Actos® (pioglitazone)
15, 30, 45 mg (TAB/CAP)

Humulin R®, Novolin R® (regular human insulin) **KEEP REFRIGERATED**
100 units/mL, 500 units/mL (injection solution)

Lantus® (insulin glargine) **KEEP REFRIGERATED**
100 units/mL (injection solution)

Glucophage® (metformin)
500, 850, 1,000 mg (TAB/CAP)
Note: metformin is also available in 500, 750, and 1,000 mg extended-release tablets.

Glucotrol® (glipizide)
5, 10 mg (TAB/CAP)
Note: glipizide is also available in a 2.5, 5, and 10 mg extended-release tablet.

Amaryl® (glimepiride)
1, 2, 4 mg (TAB/CAP)

Januvia® (sitagliptin)
25, 50, 100 mg (TAB/CAP)

Depression
Wellbutrin® (bupropion)
75, 100 mg (TAB/CAP)
Note: bupropion is also available in 100, 150, and 200 mg sustained release tablets (Wellbutrin® SR) and 150 and 300 mg extended release tablets (Wellbutrin® XL).

Remeron® (mirtazapine)
15, 30, 45 mg (TAB/CAP and ODT)

Prozac® (fluoxetine)
10, 20, 40 mg (TAB/CAP), 20 mg/5mL (oral syrup and oral solution)
Note: fluoxetine is also available in a 90 mg dose called Prozac® Weekly.

Effexor® (venlafaxine)
25, 37.5, 50, 75, 100 mg (TAB/CAP)
Note: Effexor® XR is available in 37.5, 75, and 150 mg extended release capsules.

Zoloft® (sertraline)
25, 50, 100 mg (TAB/CAP)
20 mg/mL (oral solution)

Paxil® (paroxetine)
10, 20, 30, 40 mg (TAB/CAP)
10 mg/5mL (oral suspension)
Note: paroxetine is also available in 12.5, 25, and 37.5 mg extended release tablets (Paxil® CR).

Lexapro® (escitalopram)
5, 10, 20 mg (TAB/CAP)
5 mg/5mL (oral solution)

Celexa® (citalopram)
10, 20, 40 mg (TAB/CAP)
10 mg/5mL (oral solution)

Cymbalta® (duloxetine)
20(DR), 30(DR), 60(DR) mg (TAB/CAP)

Desyrel® (trazodone) *also used to treat insomnia*
50, 100 mg (TAB/CAP)
Note: trazodone is also available in 150 mg and 300 mg extended release tablets.

Elavil® (amitriptyline)
10, 25, 50, 75, 100, 150 mg (TAB/CAP)

Asthma
AccuNeb® (albuterol inhalation solution)
0.021%, 0.042%, 0.083% (inhalation solution)

Proventil®, ProAir®, Ventolin® (albuterol inhaler)
0.09 mg/actuation (inhaler)

Singulair® (montelukast)
4, 5 mg (chewable tablet)
10 mg (TAB/CAP)
4 mg (oral packet)

Advair® (fluticasone/salmeterol)
100/50, 250/50, 500/50 mcg (inhalation disk)
45/21, 115/21, 230/21 mcg/actuation (inhaler)

Chronic Obstructive Pulmonary Disease (COPD)
Atrovent® (ipratropium inhalation solution)
0.02% (inhalation solution)
0.017 mg/actuation (inhaler)
0.03%, 0.05% (nasal spray)

Spiriva® (tiotropium capsules for inhalation)
18 mcg (inhalation capsule)

Cardiac Arrhythmias
Lanoxin® (digoxin)
0.125, 0.25 mg (TAB/CAP)
0.25 mg/mL (IV solution)

Pacerone® (amiodarone)
100, 200, 400 mg (TAB/CAP)

Blood Clot Treatment/Prevention
Heparin
10, 100, 1000, 2500, 5000, 10000, 20000 units/mL (injection solution)

Coumadin®, Jantoven® (warfarin)
1, 2, 2.5, 3, 4, 5, 6, 7.5, 10 mg (TAB/CAP)
5 mg (powder for IV solution)

Ecotrin® (aspirin) *also used for pain and fever*
81, 325, 500 mg (TAB/CAP)

Plavix® (clopidogrel)
75, 300 mg (TAB/CAP)

Lovenox® (enoxaparin)
30 mg/0.3mL, 40 mg/0.4mL, 60 mg/0.6mL, 80 mg/0.8mL, 100 mg/mL, 120 mg/0.8mL, 150 mg/mL (subcutaneous solution)

Angina/Heart Attack Prevention (Vasodilators)
Apresoline® (hydralazine)
10, 25, 50, 100 mg (TAB/CAP)
20 mg/mL (injection solution)

Imdur® (isosorbide mononitrate)
10, 20, 30(ER), 60(ER), 120(ER) mg (TAB/CAP)

Nitro-bid® transdermal ointment (nitroglycerin)
2% (transdermal ointment)

Nitro-dur® transdermal patch (nitroglycerin)
0.1, 0.2, 0.3, 0.4, 0.6, 0.8 mg/hr (transdermal patch)

Nitrostat® sublingual (nitroglycerin)
0.3, 0.4, 0.6 mg (sublingual tablet)

Hypertension (High Blood Pressure)
Dyrenium® (triamterene)
50, 100 mg (TAB/CAP)

Maxzide®, Dyazide® (hydrochlorothiazide/triamterene)
25/37.5, 25/50, 50/75 mg (TAB/CAP)

Norvasc® (amlodipine)
2.5, 5, 10 mg (TAB/CAP)

Atacand® (candesartan) 4,
8, 16, 32 mg (TAB/CAP)

Accupril® (quinapril)
5, 10, 20, 40 mg (TAB/CAP)

Avalide® (irbesartan/hydrochlorothiazide)
12.5/150, 12.5/300, 25/300 mg (TAB/CAP)

Hyzaar® (losartan/hydrochlorothiazide)
12.5/50, 12.5/100, 25/100 mg (TAB/CAP)

Inderal® (propranolol) *also commonly used for migraines*
10, 20, 40, 60, 80 mg (TAB/CAP)
Note: propranolol is also available as 60, 80, 120, and 160 mg extended
release capsules (Inderal® LA, Innopran® XL).

Avapro® (irbesartan)
75, 150, 300 mg (TAB/CAP)

Cozaar® (losartan)
25, 50, 100 mg (TAB/CAP)

Microzide® hydrochlorothiazide)
12.5, 25, 50 mg (TAB/CAP)

Cardizem®, Tiazac® (diltiazem) *also used for cardiac arrhythmias*
30, 60, 60(ER), 90, 90(ER), 120, 120(ER), 180(ER), 240(ER), 300(ER), 360(ER), 420(ER)
mg (TAB/CAP)
5 mg/mL (IV solution)

Isoptin®, Calan® (verapamil) *also used for cardiac arrhythmias*
40, 80, 100(ER), 120, 120(ER), 180(ER), 200(ER), 240(ER), 300(ER), 360(ER) mg
(TAB/CAP), 2.5 mg/mL (IV solution)

Vasotec® (enalapril)
2.5, 5, 10, 20 mg (TAB/CAP)

Benicar® (olmesartan)
5, 20, 40 mg (TAB/CAP)

Catapress® (clonidine)
0.1, 0.2, 0.3 mg (TAB/CAP), 0.1, 0.2, 0.3 mg/24-hr (transdermal patch)

Altace® (ramipril)
1.25, 2.5, 5, 10 mg (TAB/CAP)

Coreg® (carvedilol)
3.125, 6.25, 12.5, 25 mg (TAB/CAP) & 10, 20, 40, 80 mg ER (CAP/TAB)

Lasix® (furosemide) *also used to treat edema*
20, 40, 80 mg (TAB/CAP), 10 mg/mL (injection solution)

Aldactone® (spironolactone)
25, 50, 100 mg (TAB/CAP)

Nifediac®, Procardia® (nifedipine)
10, 20, 30(ER), 60(ER), 90(ER) mg (TAB/CAP)

Diovan® (valsartan)
40, 80, 160, 320 mg (TAB/CAP)

Prinivil®, Zestril® (lisinopril)
2.5, 5, 10, 20, 30, 40 mg (TAB/CAP)

Lotrel® (amlodipine/benazepril)
2.5/10, 5/10, 5/20, 5/40, 10/20, 10/40 mg (TAB/CAP)

Norvasc® (amlodipine)
2.5, 5, 10 mg (TAB/CAP)

Lopressor® (metoprolol tartrate) *also used for cardiac arrhythmias*
50, 100 mg (TAB/CAP), 1 mg/mL (injection solution)

Toprol® XL (metoprolol succinate (ER)) *also used for cardiac arrhythmias*
25, 50, 100, 200 mg (TAB/CAP)

Tenormin® (atenolol)
25, 50, 100 mg (TAB/CAP)

High Cholesterol
Niaspan® (niacin)
500 mg, 750 mg, 1,000 mg ER (TAB/CAP)

Zocor® (simvastatin)
5, 10, 20, 40, 80 mg (TAB/CAP)

Mevacor® (lovastatin)
10, 20, 40 mg (TAB/CAP)

Crestor® (rosuvastatin)
5, 10, 20, 40 mg (TAB/CAP)

Tricor® (fenofibrate)
48, 145 mg (TAB/CAP)

Pravachol® (pravastatin)
10, 20, 40, 80 mg (TAB/CAP)

Lipitor® (atorvastatin)
10, 20, 40, 80 mg (TAB/CAP)

Vytorin® (ezetemibe/simvastatin)
10/10, 10/20, 10/40, 10/80 mg (TAB/CAP)

Zetia® (ezetimibe)
10 mg (TAB/CAP)

Cardiac Arrest
AtroPen® (atropine)
various concentrations (SC, IM, IV)

Gout
Zyloprim® (allopurinol)
100, 300 mg (TAB/CAP)
various concentrations (IV)

Colcrys® (colchicine)
0.6 mg (TAB/CAP)

Prostate Cancer
Lupron® (luprolide)
various concentrations (SC, IV)

Fungal Infections
Nystop® (nystatin)
100,000 units/gram (topical powder)
Note: nystatin is also available in a 100,000 unit/mL oral suspension.

Diflucan® (fluconazole)
50, 100, 150, 200 mg (TAB/CAP)
10 mg/mL and 40 mg/mL (oral suspension)
2 mg/mL (IV)

Viral Infections
Tamiflu® (oseltamivir)
75 mg (TAB/CAP)
6 mg/mL (oral suspension)

Valtrex® (valacyclovir)
500 mg, 1 gram (TAB/CAP)

Zovirax® (acyclovir)
200, 400, 800 mg (TAB/CAP)
200mg/5mL (oral suspension)
5% (topical cream and topical ointment)

Bacterial Infections
Vancocin® (vancomycin)
125 mg, 250 mg (TAB/CAP)
various concentrations (IV)

Ery-tab® (erythromycin)
250, 333, 500(DR) mg (TAB/CAP)

Avelox® (moxifloxacin)
400 mg (TAB/CAP)
various concentrations (IV)

Penicillin (Generic Only)
250, 500 mg (TAB/CAP)
125 mg/5mL, 250 mg/5mL (oral suspension)
various concentrations (IV)

Tetracycline (Generic Only)
250, 500 mg (TAB/CAP)

Flagyl® (metronidazole)
250, 375, 500, 750 mg ER (TAB/CAP)
various concentrations (IV)

Omnicef® (cefdinir)
300 mg (TAB/CAP)
125 mg/5mL, 250 mg/5mL (oral suspension)

Vibramycin® (doxycycline)
100 mg (TAB/CAP)
25 mg/5mL, 50 mg/5mL (oral suspension)

Augmentin® (amoxicillin/clavulanate)
250/125, 500/125, 875/125, 1,000/62.5 mg ER (TAB/CAP)
125/31.25 mg/5mL, 250/62.5 mg/5mL (oral suspension)

Keflex® (cephalexin)
250, 500, 750 mg (TAB/CAP)
125 mg/5mL, 250 mg/5mL (oral suspension)

Bactrim®, Septra® (sulfamethoxazole/trimethoprim)
80/400 mg, 160/800 mg (TAB/CAP)
400/200 mg/5mL (oral suspension)

Cipro® (ciprofloxacin)
100, 250, 500, 750 mg (TAB/CAP)
250 mg/5 mL, 500 mg/5 mL (oral suspension)
10 mg/mL (IV solution)

Cleocin® (clindamycin)
75, 150, 300 mg (TAB/CAP)
6 mg/mL, 12 mg/mL, 18 mg/mL, 150 mg/mL (IV solution)
1% (Topical Gel, Jelly, Lotion, Pad, Solution, and Foam)
2% (vaginal cream), 100 mg (vaginal suppository)

Amoxil® (amoxicillin)
125, 200, 250, 400, 500, 775 ER, 875 mg (TAB/CAP)
125 mg/5mL, 200 mg/5mL, 250 mg/5mL, 400 mg/5mL (oral suspension)

Z-pak® (azithromycin)
250 mg (TAB/CAP)

Zithromax® (azithromycin)
250, 500, 600 mg (TAB/CAP)
1 gram packet, 100 mg/5mL, 200 mg/5mL (oral suspension)
500 mg (powder for IV solution)
Note: AzaSite® is azithromycin 1% ophthalmic solution.

Levaquin® (levofloxacin)
250, 500, 750 mg (TAB/CAP)
25 mg/mL (oral solution)
5 mg/mL (IV solution)

Biaxin® (clarithromycin)
250, 500 mg (TAB/CAP)
125 mg/5mL, 250 mg/5mL (oral suspension)
Note: Biaxin® XL is a 500 mg extended-release tablet.

Attention Deficit Hyperactivity Disorder (ADHD)
Ritalin® (methylphenidate) *C-II*
5, 10, 20 mg (TAB/CAP)
Note: Ritalin® LA is an extended-release capsule available in 10, 20, 30, and 40 mg strengths.

Concerta® (methylphenidate ER) *C-II*
18 (ER), 27 (ER), 36 (ER), 54 (ER) mg (TAB/CAP)

Adderall® (amphetamine/dextroamphetamine salts) *C-II*
5, 7.5, 10, 12.5, 15, 20, 30 mg (TAB/CAP)
Note: Adderall® XR is available in 5, 10, 15, 20, 25, and 30 mg strengths.

Strattera® (atomoxetine)
10, 18, 25, 40, 60, 80, 100 mg (TAB/CAP)

Provigil® (modafinil) *C-IV* *also used to treat fatigue and narcolepsy*
100, 200 mg (TAB/CAP)

Erectile Dysfunction (ED)
Viagra® (sildenafil)
25, 50, 100 mg (TAB/CAP)
Note: Revatio® (sildenafil) is used for treatment of pulmonary hypertension and is available in a 20 mg tablet and a 10 mg/12.5mL IV solution.

Levitra® (vardenafil)
2.5, 5, 10, 20 (TAB/CAP)
Note: Staxyn® (vardenafil) is available in a 10 mg orally disintegrating tablet.

Cialis® (tadalafil)
2.5, 5, 10, 20 (TAB/CAP)

Benign Prostatic Hyperplasia (BPH)
Flomax® (tamsulosin)
0.4 mg (TAB/CAP)

Hytrin® (terazosin)
2, 5, 10 mg (TAB/CAP)

Irregular Menstrual Bleeding
Provera® (medroxyprogesterone)
2.5, 5, 10 mg (TAB/CAP)

Over-the-counter (OTC) medications are drugs that are available to patients without a prescription for self-treatment of minor symptoms or diseases. Below is a list of the Top 45 OTC Medications categorized by their primary uses.

OTC Pain Medications

Brand Name	Generic Name	Other Uses
Tylenol®	Acetaminophen	Fever
Excedrin® Migraine	Acetaminophen, Aspirin, and Caffeine	Migraine Headaches
Ecotrin®	Aspirin	Fever, Prevent Blood Clot
Advil®, Motrin®	Ibuprofen	Fever, Inflammation
Aleve®	Naproxen	Fever, Inflammation
Azo®	Phenazopyridine	*Urinary Pain Only

*Azo (Phenazopyridine) is only effective in treating urinary pain/burning.

OTC Antacids

Brand Name	Generic Name
Maalox®	Aluminum Hydroxide, Magnesium Hydroxide, and Simethicone
Mylanta®	Aluminum Hydroxide, Magnesium Hydroxide, and Simethicone
Pepto-Bismol®	Bismuth Subsalicylate
Gaviscon®	Aluminum Hydroxide and Magnesium Carbonate
Alka-Seltzer®	Citric Acid and Sodium Bicarbonate
Tums®	Calcium Carbonate
Rolaids®	Calcium Carbonate and Magnesium Hydroxide
Pepcid®	Famotidine
Zantac®	Ranitidine
Tagamet®	Cimetidine
Prilosec OTC®	Omeprazole
Nexium®	Esomeprazole
Prevacid®	Lansoprazole

*Antacids are typically effective in treating symptoms like heartburn, indigestion, nausea, and upset stomach. Antacids that contain aluminum or calcium may also treat diarrhea, and antacids with simethicone work to reduce gas and bloating.

OTC Laxatives

Brand Name	Generic Name
Metamucil®	Psyllium Fiber
Citrate of Magnesium	Magnesium Citrate
Milk of Magnesia®	Magnesium Hydroxide
Colace®, Senokot®	Docusate
Senokot-S®	Docusate/Sennosides
Dulcolax®	Bisacodyl
Miralax®	Polyethylene Glycol (PEG) 3350

*All laxatives are used to treat constipation.

OTC Cough and Cold Medications

Brand Name	Generic Name	Specific Use
Delsym®	Dextromethorphan	Cough Suppressant
Robitussin®	Guaifenesin	Expectorant
Sudafed®	Pseudoephedrine	Decongestant
Afrin® Nasal Spray (NS)	Oxymetazoline	Nasal Decongestant
Neo-Synephrine® NS	Phenylephrine	Nasal Decongestant

OTC Allergy Medications (Antihistamines)

Brand Name	Generic Name
Benadryl®	Diphenhydramine
Claritin®, Alavert®	Loratadine
Zyrtec®	Cetirizine
Allegra®	Fexofenadine
Chlor-Trimeton®	Chlorpheniramine
Zaditor®, Alaway® Eye Drops	Ketotifen
Nasacort® Nasal Spray	Triamcinolone

OTC Antifungals

Brand Name	Generic Name
Lamisil®	Terbinafine
Lamisil® AF	Tolnaftate
Lotrimin®	Clotrimazole
Zeasorb®	Miconazole

*OTC antifungals are to be used for minor topical fungal infections (e.g. jock itch, athlete's foot, and ringworm).

For people without vitamin deficiencies, the best way to obtain vitamins is through a well-balanced diet of wholesome foods. There are 2 categories of vitamins: fat-soluble and water-soluble. There are 4 fat-soluble vitamins: A, D, E, and K. All other vitamins are water-soluble (all of the B vitamins and vitamin C). Excessive doses of fat-soluble vitamins (A, D, E, and K) over long periods of time can lead to toxicity and adverse effects since they accumulate in fat tissue. Excessively high doses of water-soluble vitamins are readily eliminated in the urine and generally cause fewer problems. Keep in mind that, while rare, excessively high doses of some water-soluble vitamins can still produce adverse effects; for example, excessively high doses of vitamin C can cause diarrhea.

Vitamin A (Retinol)
Uses: Needed for low-light vision.
Recommended adult dose: 2,000 – 3,000 IU/day
Max dose: 10,000 IU/day; excessive doses in pregnant women can cause birth defects.
Notes: When beta-carotene is consumed, from carrots and sweet potatoes for instance, it is converted to vitamin A inside the body.

Vitamin B1 (Thiamine)
Uses: Needed for metabolism of carbohydrates.
Recommended adult dose: 1 – 1.5 mg/day (10 mg/day for cataract prevention)
Max dose: None established.

Vitamin B2 (Riboflavin)
Uses: Needed for metabolism of fats, proteins, and carbohydrates.
Recommended adult dose: 1 mg/day
Max dose: None established.

Vitamin B3 (Niacin)
Uses: Lowers cholesterol and triglycerides.
Recommended adult dose: 14 – 18 mg/day
Max dose: 35 mg/day; excessive doses cause flushing.
Notes: Flushing can be prevented by taking an NSAID (e.g. aspirin) with the niacin.

Vitamin B5 (Pantothenic Acid)
Uses: Needed for metabolism of nutrients & synthesis of certain enzymes.
Recommended adult dose: 5 mg/day
Max Dose: None established; excessive doses can cause diarrhea.

Vitamin B6 (Pyridoxine)

Uses: Needed for metabolism, immune function, and fetal brain development.

Recommended adult dose: 1.5 mg/day

Max dose: 100 mg for adults; excessive doses can cause severe nerve damage.

Vitamin B7 (Biotin)

Uses: Needed for metabolism of nutrients; commonly used to help strengthen nails and hair.

Recommended adult dose: 30 mcg/day

Max dose: None established.

Vitamin B9 (Folic Acid)

Uses: Needed for cell development; most notably used during pregnancy to prevent fetal neural tube defects.

Recommended adult dose: 400 mcg/day (600 mcg/day for pregnant women)

Max dose: 1,000 mcg/day (higher doses may be used for certain conditions).

Vitamin B12 (Cobalamin)

Uses: Needed for DNA and red blood cell production.

Recommended adult dose: ~ 2.4 mcg/day

Max dose: None established (high doses have not been shown to be harmful).

Notes: A protein in the stomach called "intrinsic factor" is needed to absorb vitamin B12. Patients deficient in this protein become deficient in vitamin B12 and develop a condition known as "pernicious anemia." Like other types of anemia, this condition is characterized by a low red blood cell count. Metformin is a diabetes drug notorious for interfering with the body's ability to absorb vitamin B12.

Vitamin C (Ascorbic Acid)

Uses: Needed for its antioxidant properties to protect cells from free radical damage; the body also uses vitamin C in collagen production, which is needed for wound healing.

Recommended adult dose: 75 – 100 mg/day

Max dose: 2,000 mg/day; excessive doses can cause diarrhea and iron overload.

Notes: Vitamin C deficiency causes scurvy. Taking vitamin C with an iron supplement will increase the intestinal absorption of iron.

Vitamin D (Ergocalciferol (D2), Cholecalciferol (D3))

Uses: Needed for nerve function, immune function, and most notably for the absorption of dietary calcium.

Recommended adult dose: 400 – 800 IU/day

Max dose: 4,000 IU/day; excessive doses can damage kidneys and/or cause high calcium levels, leading to cardiac arrhythmias.

Notes: Vitamin D deficiency causes rickets in children and osteomalacia in adults, conditions in which the bones become brittle and soft. *Xenical® (orlistat)* and *Alli® (orlistat)* are weight-loss drugs that work by reducing intestinal absorption of fats. As a result, these drugs can lead to a deficiency in fat-soluble vitamins (A, D, E, and K).

Vitamin E (Alpha-Tocopherol and 7 other related compounds)

Uses: Needed for its antioxidant properties to protect cells from free radical damage; the body also needs vitamin E for immune function and cardiovascular health.

Recommended adult dose: 22 IU/day

Max dose: 1,100 – 1,500 IU/day; excessive doses can cause bleeding.

Notes: Vitamin E deficiency is rare but can cause nerve damage, muscle damage, and a weakened immune system. The risk for experiencing bleeding while taking vitamin E is especially high for patients on antiplatelet or anticoagulant medications like *aspirin, clopidogrel, prasugrel, rivaroxaban, warfarin,* and *heparin.*

****

A note about antioxidants

Antioxidants tend to interfere with cancer chemotherapy and radiation therapy, thus reducing the effectiveness of these cancer treatments. Why? Because antioxidants protect cells (including cancer cells) from free radicals, and oftentimes free radicals (such as radiation) are used as a form of therapy to kill cancer cells.

****

Vitamin K (Phytonadione)

Uses: Essential for blood clot formation; sometimes used topically to treat rosacea, stretch marks, scars, and burns; most notably used orally or by injection to reverse the effects of warfarin.

Recommended dose: 90 – 120 mcg/day

Max dose: None established.

Notes: Vitamin K intake should be consistent for patients using warfarin. If a patient ingests more than their normal amount of vitamin K while on warfarin, he/she would be at a higher risk for blood clots. If a patient ingests below their normal amount of vitamin K while on warfarin, he/she would be at a higher risk for bleeding.

Herbal supplements rarely have conclusive data to show that they are safe and effective in treating medical conditions. For this reason, pharmacists typically do not recommend herbal supplements to their patients; nonetheless, herbal supplements can be appropriate in some cases, and there are some patients who choose to make use of these products. Below is a list of the Top 30 Herbal Supplements and their primary uses.

Aloe: Heal burns/wounds topically and promote digestive health when ingested
Biotin: Strengthen hair and nails
Black Cohosh: Alleviate symptoms of menopause
Cinnamon: Decrease blood sugar in patients with diabetes
Coenzyme Q-10: Promote cardiovascular health
Echinacea: Boost immune system
Evening Primrose Oil: Alleviate symptoms of menopause
Feverfew: Alleviate migraine headaches
Fish Oil: Promote cardiovascular health and decrease blood triglyceride levels
Flaxseed Oil: Reduce inflammation and lower blood cholesterol levels
Folic Acid: Prevent fetal neural tube defects (taken before & during pregnancy)
Garlic: Decrease blood pressure
Ginger: Reduce nausea
Gingko: Improve memory and increase blood circulation
Glucosamine & Chondroitin: Alleviate osteoarthritis pain
Green Tea: Increase metabolism; cancer prevention (antioxidant properties)
Hoodia: Promote weight-loss
Kava Kava: Reduce symptoms of anxiety
Melatonin: Promote sleep; may be used in the treatment of insomnia
Milk Thistle: Promote liver health
Peppermint: Alleviate heartburn and upset stomach
Probiotics: Promote digestive health
Red Yeast Rice: Lower blood cholesterol levels
St. John's Wort: Improve depression (this supplement has *many* drug interactions)
SAM-e: Stabilize mood
Saw Palmetto: Reduce prostate size in patients with BPH
Senna: Stimulate bowel movements
Valerian: Promote sleep and reduce symptoms of anxiety
Witch Hazel: Treat various skin conditions
Yohimbe: Treat erectile dysfunction (this supplement can raise blood pressure)

Combination drug are formulations containing two or more active ingredients. These are 20 commonly prescribed combination drugs that did not make the Top 238 Prescription Drugs list. I added them because they can be a real killer on the exam. After all, you either know them or you don't.

Aggrenox® (aspirin/dipyridamole) – Blood clot prevention
Benicar® HCT (olmesartan/hydrochlorothiazide) – High blood pressure
Benzaclin® (benzoyl peroxide/clindamycin) – Acne (topical)
Fioricet® (acetaminophen/caffeine/butalbital) – Migraine headaches
Glucovance® (glyburide/metformin) – Diabetes
Hyzaar® (losartan/hydrochlorothiazide) – High blood pressure
Jalyn® (dutasteride/tamsulosin) – Enlarged prostate (BPH)
Janumet® (sitagliptin/metformin) – Diabetes
Kaletra® (lopinavir/ritonavir) – HIV/AIDS
Lotrel® (amlodipine/benazepril) – High blood pressure
Metaglip® (glipizide/metformin) – Diabetes
Sinemet® (carbidopa/levodopa) – Parkinson's disease
Stalevo® (carbidopa/levodopa/entacapone) – Parkinson's disease
Symbyax® (olanzapine/fluoxetine) – Depression in bipolar disorder
Tenoretic® (atenolol/chlorthalidone) – High blood pressure
Tobradex® (tobramycin/dexamethasone) – Bacterial infections of the eye
Tribenzor® (olmesartan/amlodipine/hydrochlorothiazide) – High blood pressure
Vicoprofen® (ibuprofen/hydrocodone) – Pain and inflammation
Vimovo® (naproxen/esomeprazole) – Arthritis pain and stomach acid
Zegerid® (omeprazole/sodium bicarbonate) – GERD

Note: blood pressure medications are commonly formulated as combination drugs. This is because most patients with hypertension need more than one medication to achieve adequate blood pressure control.

What is the benefit of having two or more active ingredients in one capsule or tablet?
One of the biggest challenges prescribers and pharmacists face is getting patients to consistently take their medications exactly as prescribed. When a patient consistently remembers to take their medication as prescribed, the patient is considered to be *compliant* (or *"adherent"*). When the patient frequently misses doses of medication, the patient is considered to be *non-compliant* (or *"non-adherent"*). Patients may lack consistency due to forgetfulness, lack of education regarding the benefits of therapy, and/or an inability to afford the medication. By supplying two or more active ingredients in one capsule or tablet, the patient now only has to remember to take one tablet or capsule instead of two. This has a positive impact on patient compliance.

When trying to determine the function of a drug, sometimes you will find a clue in the drug name itself. These clues are called "drug name stems" and they appear in the generic names of certain drugs. Below are some examples:

-afil = phosphodiesterase 5 (PDE-5) inhibitor (e.g. tadalafil, sildenafil, vardenafil) used to treat erectile dysfunction and/or pulmonary arterial hypertension.

-azepam or **-azolam** = benzodiazepine (e.g. alprazolam, clonazepam, oxazepam, diazepam) used to treat anxiety and/or insomnia.

-azole = antifungal (e.g. clotrimazole, ketoconazole) used to treat fungal infections.

-barbital = barbiturate or barbiturate derivatrive (e.g. phenobarbital, pentobarbital, secobarbital, amobrbital) used to treat anxiety, insomnia, and/or seizures.

Ceph- or **Cef-** = cephalosporin antibiotic (e.g. cephalexin, cefazolin, ceftriaxone, ceftazidime, cefdinir) used to treat bacterial infections.

-dronate = bisphosphonate (e.g. ibandronate, alendronate, risedronate) used to treat or prevent osteoporosis.

-floxacin = fluoroquinolone antibiotic (e.g. ciprofloxacin, moxifloxacin, levofloxacin) used to treat bacterial infections.

-gliptin = dipeptidyl peptidase 4 (DPP-4) inhibitor (e.g. saxagliptin, sitagliptin, linagliptin) used to lower blood sugar in type II diabetes mellitus.

-icillin = penicillin antibiotic (e.g. penicillin, amoxicillin, ampicillin, methicillin) used to treat bacterial infections.

-isone = corticosteroid (e.g. prednisone, methylprednisone, hydrocortisone) used to suppress the immune system and reduce inflammation.

-olol = bet-blocker (e.g. metoprolol, atenolol, propranolol, bisoprolol) used to lower blood pressure and/or treat other cardiac conditions such as arrhythmias.

-osin = alpha adrenergic receptor blocker (α-blocker) (e.g. doxazosin, terazosin, prazosin, tamsulosin) used to treat high blood pressure and/or benign prostatic hyperplasia (BPH).

-prazole = proton pump inhibitor (PPI) (e.g. omeprazole, lansoprazole, pantoprazole, rabeprazole) used to suppress stomach acid production.

-pril = angiotensin converting enzyme inhibitor (ACEI) (e.g. lisinopril, benazepril) used to lower blood pressure.

-sartan = angiotensin receptor blocker (ARB) (e.g. valsartan, losartan, olmesartan) used to reduce blood pressure.

-setron = 5-HT$_3$ (serotonin) antagonist (e.g. ondansetron, palonosetron, granisetron) used to treat or prevent nausea and vomiting (especially nausea and vomiting associated with cancer chemotherapy).

-statin = HMG-CoA reductase inhibitor (e.g. atorvastatin, simvastatin, lovastatin, pravastatin) used to lower cholesterol.

-tidine = H2 receptor blockers (e.g. ranitidine, famotidine, cimetidine) used to suppress stomach acid production.

-triptan = serotonin agonist (5-HT agonist) (e.g. sumatriptan, zolmitriptan, naratriptan, eletriptan) used to treat migraine headaches.

-vir = antiviral (e.g. ritonavir, lopinavir, acyclovir, valacyclovir) used to treat viral infections like shingles, genital herpes, and HIV/AIDS.

There are four major types of drug interactions: drug-drug, drug-supplement, drug-food, and drug-disease. Below you will find a list of the most common drug interactions.

Common Drug-Drug Interactions

Warfarin and NSAIDs*

Warfarin is an anticoagulant used to prevent or treat blood clots. A major side effect of warfarin is bleeding. NSAIDs are notorious for damaging the lining of the stomach, which has the potential to lead to a gastrointestinal bleed. When warfarin and NSAIDs are used together, the risk of a life-threatening GI bleed increases significantly. NSAIDs also have some "anti-platelet" (blood-thinning) effect, which further increases bleed risk. *Some examples of generic NSAIDs include: Ibuprofen, Naproxen, Aspirin, Meloxicam, Indomethacin, and Diclofenac.

Warfarin and Antibiotics

Antibiotics increase the bleeding risk associated with warfarin. The reason for this is explained below.

How Warfarin Works
The body uses Vitamin K to activate the "vitamin K-dependent clotting factors" (factors 2, 7, 9, and 10). Once vitamin K is used to activate a clotting factor, it is deactivated, rendered incapable of activating more clotting factors unless it is reactivated by the enzyme "Vitamin K Epoxide Reductase Complex 1" (VKORC1). Warfarin inhibits VKORC1, thus preventing activation of vitamin K-dependent clotting factors. In simpler terms, warfarin reduces blood clotting by keeping vitamin K in its deactivated form. Since vitamin K is deactivated, it cannot activate certain clotting factors.

Why Antibiotics Interact with Warfarin
Vitamin K enters the body from two sources: the diet (e.g. green leafy vegetables, mayonnaise) and intestinal flora (normal bacteria that reside in the intestine). Intestinal flora produces vitamin K, which gets absorbed into the bloodstream. When antibiotics are introduced into the body, some of the intestinal flora is killed. Since there are fewer bacteria producing vitamin K in the intestine, less vitamin K enters the bloodstream from that source. This results in an exaggerated effect of warfarin, potentially leading to over-anticoagulation and bleeding.

Oral Contraceptives and Antibiotics

Antibiotics can decrease the effect of oral contraceptives, which increases the likelihood of contraceptive failure and increases risk of pregnancy. The prevailing theory behind this interaction is reduced enterohepatic circulation of estrogen caused by antibiotic-induced reduction of intestinal flora.

Enterohepatic Circulation of Estrogen

Some estrogen is eliminated by excretion into the bile where is is carried out of the body during defecation. Some of the estrogen that goes into the bile gets hydrolyzed by intestinal flora and subsequently reabsorbed into the blood where it is given another opportunity to exert its pharmacologic effect. Since antibiotics kill intestinal flora, less estrogen gets hydrolyzed and reabsorbed (i.e. the effect of estrogen is reduced).

Nitrates and PDE-5 Inhibitors

Both of these drugs dilate blood vessels. When taken together, blood pressure can drop to a dangerously low level. PDE-5 inhibitors include: Viagra® (sildenafil), Levitra® (vardenafil), and Cialis® (tadalafil).

Lithium and Diuretics

Lithium is used as a mood stabilizer in psychiatric disorders, and it can also be used to treat/prevent migraine headaches. Lithium is considered to be a "narrow therapeutic index drug," which means that there is less than a 2-fold difference between the median lethal dose and the median effective dose, or there is less than a 2-fold difference between the minimum toxic concentration and the minimum effective concentration. In other words, if the concentration of the drug in the blood gets too high, this therapeutic agent becomes a deadly toxin. The kidneys, which act as a filtration system for the blood, take lithium from the blood so it can leave the body in the urine. Diuretics work by causing the kidneys to transfer more than normal amounts of sodium and water from the blood into the urine. When more sodium is filtered out of the blood by the kidneys, a higher-than-normal amount of lithium is absorbed from the urine back into the blood. As a result, when taking diuretics while on lithium therapy, the concentration of lithium in the blood increases. This can lead to lithium toxicity and, in severe cases, death.

Phenytoin and Macrolide Antibiotics

Phenytoin is an anticonvulsant drug (used to treat/prevent seizures). Phenytoin is also a narrow therapeutic index drug. Enzymes in liver metabolize and deactivate phenytoin. Macrolide antibiotics (clarithromycin, azithromycin, and erythromycin) and certain other drugs block the key enzymes in the liver responsible for metabolizing and deactivating phenytoin. When a person takes macrolide antibiotics while on phentyoin, this results in elevated concentrations of phenytoin in the blood. In severe cases, the result can be lethal.

Common Drug-Supplement Interactions

St. John's Wort and CYP3A4 Substrates

St. John's Wort induces the production of enzyme CYP3A4. This enzyme is important, as it is involved in the metabolism of approximately 50% of all drugs. Induction of CYP3A4 leads to the deactivation of drugs that are substrates of CYP3A4. Examples include oral contraceptives, HIV protease inhibitors, carbamazepine, colchicine, cyclosporine, dexamethasone, and methylprednisolone.

Garlic and CYP3A4 Substrates

Garlic has an effect similar to St. John's Wort; it induces CYP3A4.

Cations* and Levothyroxine, Quinolones, Tetracyclines, and Bisphosphonates

These drugs can chelate (i.e. bind to) divalent cations (e.g. magnesium (Mg^{2+}), calcium (Ca^{2+})) and trivalent cations (e.g. iron (Fe^{3+}), aluminum (Al^{3+})) in the gut, leading to precipitation (solidification) of the drug-ion complex. The precipitated drug never gets absorbed, but passes through the GI tract, never getting the opportunity to exert its pharmacologic effect.

*Only polyvalent cations, not monovalent ions such as Na^+ and K^+. Remember a *cation* is a positively charged ion, and an *anion* is a negatively charged ion.

Ginkgo and NSAIDs, Anticoagulants, or Anti-platelets*

Ginkgo has anti-platelet effects. When combined with other drugs that have an inhibitory effect on blood clotting, the risk of bleeding is increased.

*Anti-platelets include drugs like clopidogrel and prasugrel.

Dong Quai and NSAIDs, Anticoagulants, or Anti-platelets

Dong Quai is primarily used to treat PMS, menstrual cramps, and symptoms of menopause. It contains chemicals known as "coumarin derivatives;" notice how the name "coumarin" is similar to Coumadin®? Coumarin derivatives, like warfarin, are vitamin K antagonists, so it is not surprising that dong quai increases the risk of bleeding when taken with other drugs that inhibit blood clotting.

Fish Oil and NSAIDs, Anticoagulants, or Anti-platelets

At doses greater than 3 grams/day, fish oil can increase the risk of bleeding. Not surprisingly, the risk of bleeding is significantly higher when fish oil is taken with other drugs that increase the risk of bleeding.

Common Drug-Food Interactions

HMG-CoA Reductase Inhibitors (Statins) and Grapefruit Juice

> Grapefruit juice inhibits the enzyme CYP3A4, a major enzyme involved in the metabolism of certain statins. This elevates the statin levels to higher than normal, leading to increased risk of rhabdomyolysis.

Levodopa and Protein

> Levodopa is used to treat symptoms of Parkinson's Disease. Dietary protein (e.g. from meat, nuts, and dairy products) interferes with the intestinal absorption of levodopa. Proteins also interfere with levodopa crossing the blood-brain barrier, which levodopa must cross to reach its site of action. As a result, when levodopa is taken with a high protein meal, less levodopa reaches the site of action (the brain).

Warfarin and Foods High in Vitamin K*

> Since warfarin interferes with the activity of vitamin K, warfarin's effect can be reduced if dietary vitamin K intake increases. As a general rule, patients on warfarin should not avoid vitamin K but should make an effort to be consistent in how much vitamin K they consume each day. *Foods high in vitamin K include: spinach, kale, collard greens, turnip greens, broccoli, Brussels sprouts, mayonnaise, green tea, and canola oil.

> Note: Some multivitamins contain vitamin K.

Monoamine Oxidase Inhibitors (MAOI)* and Foods/Beverages Rich in Tyramine**

> Tyramine is a monoamine that stimulates catecholamine release in the body. Catecholamines (e.g. epinephrine, norepinephrine) are vasopressors – they increase blood pressure. When the enzyme monoamine oxidase is inhibited, tyramine is not eliminated. As a result, tyramine builds up as it is consumed, leading to massive release of catecholamines and hypertensive crisis (potentially fatal).

> *Monoamine Oxidase Inhibitors (MAOIs) include: Tranylcypromine, Phenelzine, and Selegiline.

> **Foods/beverages rich in tyramine include: most things that are smoked, aged, pickled, or fermented (e.g. aged cheeses, aged meats, wines), chocolate, licorice, tofu, soy sauce, avocados, and bananas.

Common Drug-Disease Interactions

Decongestants* and Hypertension

When sinus blood vessels are swollen and large, they leak fluid and cause sinus congestion. Decongestants provide relief by constricting blood vessels. The blood vessels that are constricted by decongestants are not limited to those located in the sinus passages. Decongestants constrict blood vessels all throughout the body, leading to increased blood pressure. In severe cases, use of a decongestant by an individual with hypertension could result in a cardiovascular event (e.g. stroke, aneurism).

*Decongestants include: Sudafed® (pseudoephedrine) and Sudafed® PE (phenylephrine).

Aspirin and Peptic Ulcer Disease

Aspirin has an anti-platelet effect, which predisposes patients to bleeding. This drug is also notorious from causing damage to the lining of the stomach. Patients with peptic ulcer disease have lesions in the lining of their stomach. These lesions can be irritated by aspirin, potentially leading to a gastrointestinal bleed.

NSAIDs and Chronic Renal Failure

NSAIDs decrease prostaglandin production. Prostaglandins promote renal blood flow. Less prostaglandin leads to less renal blood flow. Less blood flow leads to additional renal impairment.

TCAs* and Dementia

Tricyclic antidepressants (TCAs) have anti-cholinergic effects. Dementia is theorized to result from an imbalance between two neurotransmitters (acetylcholine and dopamine). When a patient with dementia takes a drug with anti-cholinergic properties, the imbalance and the degree of dementia can worsen.

Solution – made up of a solute and a solvent; the solute molecules dissolve into a homogenous, single-phase mixture with the solvent.

Syrup – Highly concentrated water-based sugar solutions.
Example: Simple Syrup (85%(w/v) solution of sucrose in water).

Elixir – Solutions containing water, alcohol, and sweetener.
Example: Lortab® Elixir.

Tincture – Usually alcoholic extracts of crude materials.
Example: Tincture of opium is derived from the poppy plant (*Papaver somniferum*) – a crude (i.e. raw) material.

Suspension – a mixture of particles (could be solid or fluid) dispersed in a fluid; the particles do not dissolve, the mixture is two-phase.*

Emulsion – a suspension of two immiscible liquids (two liquids that will not dissolve in one another as they would in a solution).
Example: Oil in water.

*Two-phase mixtures (e.g. suspensions/emulsions) must be shaken to ensure that the patient is receiving the correct amount of medication in each dose; you should place a label on the prescription bottle that says "shake well." For instance, look at the image below. Imagine that the drug is represented by the gray phase. If the mixture is not shaken, the patient will receive too little of the gray phase (the drug) in the first few doses and too much of the gray phase (the drug) in the last few doses.

Illustration: *Why Suspensions Must Be Shaken*

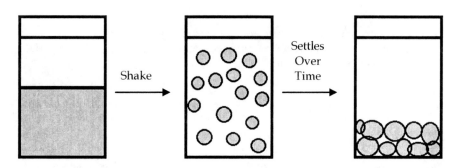

Tablets
A powdery mixture of an active pharmaceutical ingredient and excipients (inert/inactive ingredients, sometimes referred to as "fillers") pressed into a disc or other small shape. Many, if not most, drugs are available in tablet form.

****

Scored Tablets
Certain tablets should never be split or crushed. For instance, most extended-release tablets and capsules *must* be swallowed whole because splitting or crushing can destroy the slow release mechanism and cause overdosing. On the other hand, some tablets are designed by the manufacturer with an indentation (i.e. they are "scored") to make it easy for the patient to divide the tablet into halves or quarters. Below is an illustration of two scored tablets. On the left we see a tablet that is scored into equal quarters and on the right we see a tablet that is scored into equal halves. Below each tablet is an illustration of the side view (each tablet rotated 90 degrees on the dashed-line axis) – note the indentation.

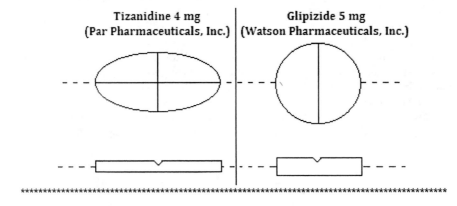

| Tizanidine 4 mg (Par Pharmaceuticals, Inc.) | Glipizide 5 mg (Watson Pharmaceuticals, Inc.) |

****

Capsules
Capsules are made up of two parts: the shell (usually made of gelatin or cellulose) and the contents (may be drug powder, pellets, small tablets, or liquid). Many drugs are available in capsule form

Caplets
Caplets are capsule-shaped tablets.

Enteric Coated (EC) Tablets
These tablets are coated with a special material (enteric coating) that will not dissolve in the acidic environment of the stomach but will dissolve in the less acidic environment inside the small intestines. As a result, when enteric coated tablets are ingested, they do not dissolve until they reach the intestine. This type of coating is typically used for medications that can irritate the lining of the stomach. A great example is enteric coated aspirin.

Sublingual (SL) Tablets

These tablets dissolve under the tongue and deliver the drug across the tissue beneath the tongue and directly into the bloodstream. By entering the bloodstream directly, the drug can exert is pharmacologic effect much more quickly. This method of administration also avoids first-pass metabolism (see section on routes of administration for further detail). A great example is the nitroglycerin sublingual tablet.

Orally Disintegrating Tablets (ODT)

These tablets dissolve in the saliva; no water is required when taking an ODT. They are especially useful in patients that experience difficulty or pain when swallowing. For example, let's say a patient has experienced severe nausea and vomiting. The stomach acid from the vomit has damaged the lining of the patient's esophagus, making it extremely painful to swallow. To avoid swallowing, the patient can use an ondansetron ODT (used to treat nausea) instead of regular ondansetron tablets.

Lozenges

These medicated tablets or candies are designed to dissolve slowly – and thus release medication slowly – to a location within the oral cavity. An example of a medicated candy lozenge is the Cepacol® Sore Throat Lozenge, which delivers benzocaine and menthol directly to the site of pain in the throat. Clotrimazole is another example, which is available as a tablet lozenge for the treatment of oral thrush.

> **Note:** A "troche" is technically a compressed lozenge, but many people use the terms "lozenge" and "troche" synonymously.

How do you determine that a generic drug is equivalent to a brand drug?
It is listed as an A-rated drug in the Federal Orange Book.

What is the official title for the Orange Book?
Approved Drug Products with Therapeutic Equivalence Evaluations

True or false. A drug with a narrow therapeutic index is never considered to be generically equivalent to the brand name product.
True.

A prescription for Lipitor® is given to you verbally over the telephone. Should you dispense the brand name Lipitor or the generic equivalent atorvastatin?
Atorvastatin. You would only dispense the brand name if the prescriber (or his/her agent) expressly says that the brand name is necessary and substitution is not allowed.

What is a narrow therapeutic index drug?
A drug that requires careful dose titration and patient monitoring in order to be used safely and effectively. One of the two following criteria must apply:

- There is less than a 2-fold difference between the median lethal dose (LD50) and the median effective dose (ED50).
- There is less than a 2-fold difference between the minimum toxic concentration (MTC) and the minimum effective concentration (MEC).

Note: ED50 is the dose that produces the desired effect in 50% of the population using the drug, and LD 50 is the dose that is lethal in 50% of the population using the drug.

Does the FDA publish a current list of NTI drugs?
No.

KNOWLEDGE DOMAIN #2
PHARMACY LAW AND REGULATIONS
(12.5% OF EXAM)

State Board of Pharmacy
Each state has its own board of pharmacy that is responsible for protecting the health, safety, and welfare of its citizens in matters involving the practice of pharmacy. This is accomplished by enforcing of pharmacy laws and regulations. State boards of pharmacy are also in charge of regulating traditional compounding pharmacies.

Food and Drug Administration (FDA)
The FDA enforces drug manufacturing laws and regulates prescription drug advertising, which is known as "direct to consumer" (DTC) advertising. The FDA also regulates large-scale compounding facilities.

Drug Enforcement Agency (DEA)
The DEA enforces the federal Controlled Substances Act (CSA) and makes decisions regarding the classification of certain drugs as controlled substances.

Occupational Safety and Health Administration (OSHA)
OSHA enforces health and safety laws. They play a major role in enforcing measures to reduce the risk of employee exposure to bloodborne pathogens. This is particularly relevant to pharmacies that compound infusions and/or administer vaccinations (i.e. pharmacies that work with needles).

Federal Trade Commission (FTC)
The FTC regulates over-the-counter drug, medical device, cosmetic, and food advertising.

> **Note:** Vitamins and herbal supplements are considered "food" in the eyes of the law.

What is a "misbranded" drug?

Many things can be construed as misbranding. Some definitive examples of misbranding include:

- False or misleading labeling.
- Legally noncompliant packaging/labeling.
- Unclear wording is present on the label.
- Inadequate directions for use.
- Drug use poses a danger if used as prescribed.
- Generic name is not displayed in a font size that is at least half as large as the brand name font size.

What is an "adulterated" drug?

An adulterated drug is one that has a different quality, strength, or purity than that which is stated on the label.

What characteristics define each schedule of controlled substances?

Schedule I Controlled Substance (e.g. GHB, Heroin)
- No accepted medical use.
- High potential for abuse.
- Lacks safety.

Schedule II Controlled Substance (e.g. Morphine, Codeine)
- Accepted medical use.
- High potential for abuse.
- High potential for physical/psychological dependence.

Schedule III Controlled Substance (e.g. Testosterone, Dronabinol)
- Accepted medical use.
- Moderate potential for abuse.
- Moderate-low potential for physical/psychological dependence.

Schedule IV Controlled Substance (e.g. Diazepam, Modafinil)
- Accepted medical use.
- Mild potential for abuse.
- Mild potential for physical/psychological dependence.

Schedule V Controlled Substance (e.g. Pregabalin, Lacosamide)
- Accepted medical use.
- Low potential for abuse.
- Low potential for physical/psychological dependence.

It is important to be able to recognize the schedule to which a controlled substance belongs. Below is a list of some of the most commonly known and/or used controlled substances categorized by schedule. Although some students find that certain drugs are scheduled differently in their state, the PTCB exam will test your knowledge of federal law and regulations. Your knowledge of state law will not be tested. This information was derived from the federal Controlled Substances Act. Generic names are listed with brand names in parenthesis.

Schedule I Controlled Substances

- GHB
- Heroin
- LSD
- Marijuana (**Note:** used medically in some states, but not legal for medical use according to *federal* law)
- MDMA

Schedule II Controlled Substances

C-II Opioids:
- codeine
- hydrocodone*
- morphine (MS Contin®, Kadian®, Roxanol®)
- meperidine (Demerol®)
- methadone (Dolophine®, Methadose®)
- fentanyl (Duragesic®)
- hydromorphone (Dilaudid®, Exalgo®)
- oxycodone (Roxicodone®, Oxycontin®)
- oxymorphone (Opana®)
*Effective as of October 6, 2014, this includes all hydrocodone combination products (e.g. Norco®, Lortab®, Vicodin®, Vicoprofen®, Tussionex®).

C-II Stimulants:
- amphetamine/dextroamphetamine (Adderall®)
- cocaine
- methamphetamine (Desoxyn®)
- methylphenidate (Concerta®, Metadate®, Methylin®, Ritalin®)

C-II Depressants:
- amobarbital (Amytal®)
- pentobarbital (Nembutal®)
- secobarbital (Seconal®)

C-II Hallucinogens:
- nabilone (Cesamet®)

Schedule III Controlled Substances

C-III Opioids:
- buprenorphine (Buprenex®, Subutex®)
- buprenorphine/naloxone (Suboxone®)
- camphorated tincture of opium (Paregoric®)
- codeine* (e.g. Tylenol #3, Fioricet with codeine)

*Categorized as a C-III controlled when used in limited quantities *in combination with other medications.*

C-III Mixed Opioid Agonist/Antagonists:
- nalorphine (Nalline®)

C-III Stimulants:
- benzphetamine (Didrex®, Regimex)
- phendimetrazine (Bontril®)

C-III Depressants:
- barbituric acid and its derivatives
- ketamine (Ketalar®)

These depressants that would otherwise belong to Schedule II are considered Schedule III when they exist in a compound, mixture, or suppository form
- amobarbital
- pentobarbital
- secobarbital

C-III Anabolic Steroids:
All anabolic steroids are C-III according to federal law
- testosterone (AndroGel®, Testim®, Axiron®, Depo-Testosterone®)
- oxandrolone (Oxandrin®)

C-III Hallucinogens:
- dronabinol (Marinol®)

Schedule IV Controlled Substances

<u>C-IV Depressants (Benzodiazepines):</u>
Note: All prescription benzodiazepines are federally classified as Schedule IV. The best way to recognize a benzodiazepine is by the last part of its generic name. The generic name almost always ends in "-epam" or "-olam." Below is a list of benzodiazepines. Exceptions to the naming rule are described.

- alprazolam (Xanax®)
- chlordiazepoxide (Librium®)
  - o   The first benzodiazepine formally discovered
  - o   The only benzodiazepine that ends in -epoxide.
- clonazepam (Klonopin®)
- clorazepate (Tranxene®)
  - o   One of two benzodiazepines that end in -ate.
  - o   The -aze- is another way to tell by the name that this drug is a benzodiazepine.
- diazepam (Valium®, Diastat®)
- estazolam (Prosom®)
- flurazepam (Dalmane®)
- lorazepam (Ativan®)
- midazolam (Versed®)
- temazepam (Restoril®)

<u>C-IV Depressants:</u>
- eszopiclone (Lunesta®)
- zaleplon (Sonata®)
- zolpidem (Ambien®)
- phenobarbital (Luminal®)
- carisoprodol (Soma®)
- tramadol (Ultram®)

<u>C-IV Mixed Opioid Agonist/Antagonists:</u>
- butorphanol (Stadol®)
- pentazocine (Talwin®)

<u>C-IV Stimulants:</u>
- modafinil (Provigil®)
- phentermine (Adipex-P®, Suprenza®)
- phentermine/topiramate (Qsymia®)
- sibutramine (Meridia®)

Schedule V Controlled Substances

<u>C-V Opioids:</u>
When the strength per unit dose is very small, these medications are classified as Schedule V.
- codeine (Robitussin® AC)
- diphenoxylate with atropine (Lomotil®)

<u>C-V Depressants:</u>
- pregabalin (Lyrica®)
- lacosamide (Vimpat®)

For the complete list of controlled substances, go to:
<http://www.deadiversion.usdoj.gov/schedules/orangebook/e_cs_sched.pdf>

True or false. Schedule I controlled substances can be dispensed pursuant to a valid, hand-signed prescription.
False, these drugs have no accepted medical use and cannot be prescribed.

In what setting might you find Schedule I controlled substances?
The only setting in which a Schedule I controlled substance can be legally utilized is in a legitimate research laboratory registered with the DEA.

True or false. Schedule II controlled substance prescription records can be stored in the same file as other prescription medications.
False, Schedule II prescription records must be stored separate from all other prescription records.

After an initial inventory of controlled substances has been taken (e.g. when the pharmacy initially opens to the public for business), how frequently must an inventory of controlled substances be conducted?
At least every two years.

When taking an inventory of controlled substances, does the law require you to account for drug samples?
Yes, drug samples that contain controlled substances must be accounted for in the inventory record.

According to the federal Controlled Substances Act (CSA), how should you store Schedule III – V prescription files?
Either separately from all other prescription records, or in such a way that they are readily retrievable from the non-controlled prescription records (e.g. Schedule III – V prescription records can be stored along with non-controlled substance prescription records if each controlled substance prescription is marked with the letter "C" in red ink).

When Schedule II controlled substances are sent to a reverse distributor because they are expired, damaged, or otherwise unusable, what form should be used?
DEA Form 222.

Who would be responsible for filling out the Form 222?
The reverse distributor – the entity receiving the substance is always the one that fills out the form.

When Schedule III – V controlled substances are returned, is a DEA Form 222 necessary?
No, Schedule III – V controlled substances may be transferred via invoice (DEA Form 222 is only used for Schedule I and II controlled substances).

How long must the pharmacy keep controlled substance return records, prescription records, and inventory records?
2 years.

What information must be included on a controlled substance prescription?
1. Patient's full name
2. Patient's address
3. Prescriber's full name
4. Prescribers work address
5. Prescriber's DEA number
6. Drug name
7. Drug strength
8. Dosage form
9. Quantity prescribed
10. Directions for use
11. Number of refills authorized (if any)

True or false. Federal law prohibits e-prescribing of C-II drugs.
False, federal law permits e-prescribing of C-II through C-V drugs; however, the software used by the prescriber sending the prescription and the pharmacy receiving the prescription must be certified by the DEA.

According to federal law, C-II prescriptions must be filled within how many days after being signed by the prescriber?
Federal law places no time limit within which a C-II prescription must be filled (i.e. the prescription is considered legally valid for an unlimited period of time after it is issued). Note, however, that many states have a law that does set a time limit.

True or false. For controlled substance prescriptions, the maximum quantity that can be dispensed according to federal law is a 30-day supply.
False, although some states and some insurance companies may limit controlled substance quantities to a 30-day supply, there are no specific federal limits.
Note: Remember that when federal and state laws differ, you must follow the more stringent of the two laws.

Are verbal orders (i.e. called in by the prescriber, no prescriber-signed prescription hard copy) for C-II prescriptions permitted?
Only in emergency situations (as determined by the pharmacist).
Note: quantity prescribed must be limited to the amount adequate to treat the patient for the duration of the emergency period.

After calling in an emergency C-II prescription, what must the prescriber do next?
Provide the pharmacy with a written and signed hard copy, which the pharmacy files away with the verbal order.

When emergency C-II prescriptions are called in, a prescriber has how many days to furnish the pharmacy with a written and signed prescription?
7 days according to federal law (your state's law may be more stringent).

True or false. Refills for C-II prescriptions are legally permitted up to 5 refills in 6 months.
False, refills for C-II prescriptions are legally prohibited.

Are C-II prescriptions received by facsimile (fax machine) considered valid?
A pharmacy can use a faxed copy of a C-II prescription to fill a prescription, but before that prescription can be dispensed the *original signed prescription* must be presented to the pharmacist.

What are the three exceptions that allow for C-II facsimile prescriptions to serve as the original prescription for recordkeeping purposes?
1. The prescription is being compounded for *home infusion*.
2. The prescription is for a patient in a *long-term care facility*.
3. The prescription is for a patient enrolled in a *hospice care program*.

A patient presents 6 prescriptions for Adderall 5 mg. Each prescription is written for 30 tablets with the instructions to take 1 tablet by mouth every morning and 1 tablet by mouth every afternoon at 3 PM. The situation appears suspicious since the patient has 6 prescriptions for Adderall. Is it even legal for the patient to have this many prescriptions for a C-II drug?
While it may be worth verifying the prescriptions with the prescriber before dispensing, federal law permits prescribers to issue a patient multiple C-II prescriptions at one time *as long as the total days' supply does not exceed 90 days*.
Note: these prescriptions would need to have the earliest fill date written on them (e.g. "do not fill until 4/15," "do not fill until 4/30," etc.).

Prescriptions for C-III, C-IV, and C-V controlled substances can be issued by what means?
• Orally.
• In writing.
• By facsimile.
• Electronically (e-prescribing) where state laws permit.

Are refills legally permissible for C-III, C-IV, and C-V prescriptions?
Yes, for C-III and C-IV drugs there can be up to 5 refills within 6 months of the date issued. Refill limitations do not apply for C-V prescriptions.

For non-controlled substance prescriptions, a prescriber's agent (e.g. nurse or secretary) may call in a verbal prescription. Is a prescriber's agent allowed to call in Schedule III – V prescriptions?
No, the individual prescriber must personally make the call to submit a C-III through V prescription verbally.

Is the individual prescriber required to personally send the fax when a C-III through V prescription is being submitted by facsimile?
No, faxes for C-III through V prescriptions may be sent by a prescriber's agent.

Can a prescriber post-date a prescription for a controlled substance (e.g. record the date of issuance as 8/14 when he/she actually wrote the prescription in 8/12)?
No. The prescriber might try to do this when he/she doesn't want the patient to have the prescription filled until 8/14, but the proper approach is to record the written date as 8/12 and write on the face of the prescription "do not fill until 8/14."

Can a controlled substance be delivered or shipped to an individual in another country if there is a valid prescription for the substance?
No, this type of exportation of a controlled substance is prohibited by the federal controlled substance act.

Prescribers that want to prescribe Schedule III – V controlled substances for treatment of narcotic addiction (i.e. buprenorphine drug products) must display what piece of additional information on the face of the prescription?
Their unique DEA registration identification number that begins with an "X" must be displayed, which is granted to prescribers that have obtained the necessary waiver* from the DEA (in addition to their standard DEA registration number).

*Typically, controlled substances used to treat narcotic addiction can only be prescribed, administered, and/or dispensed within a Narcotic Treatment Facility (NTF), but the DEA can grant a waiver to a prescriber to allow him/her to prescribe, administer, and/or dispense C-III through V drugs for treatment of narcotic addiction outside of a NTF.

What should be done in the event that theft or loss of a controlled substance is discovered?
The DEA should be notified upon discovery, and a DEA Form 106 should be filled out to document the theft or loss.

Summary of Federal Controlled Substance Act Requirements

	Schedule II	Schedule III & IV	Schedule V
DEA Registration	Required	Required	Required
Receiving Records	DEA Form 222	Invoices, Readily Retrievable	Invoices, Readily Retrievable
Prescriptions	Written Prescription*	Written, Oral, or Faxed Prescriptions	Written, Oral, Faxed, or Over The Counter**
Refills	No	No more than 5 within 6 months	As authorized when prescription is issued
Distribution Between Registrants	DEA Form 222	Invoices	Invoices
Theft or Significant Loss	Report and complete DEA Form 106	Report and complete DEA Form 106	Report and complete DEA Form 106

Note: All records must be maintained for 2 years according to federal law.
* Emergency prescriptions require a signed follow-up prescription. Exceptions: facsimile prescriptions serve as the original prescription when issued for residents of long-term care facilities, hospice patients, or patients receiving the prescribed narcotic medication as a compounded product for home infusion.
** Where authorized by state law.

What is the DEA Form 224 used for?
Applying for pharmacy DEA registration.

How frequently does a pharmacy's DEA registration need to be renewed?
Every 3 years.

What is the DEA Form 222 used for?
Ordering Schedule I and Schedule II controlled substances.

If you make a mistake when filling out a DEA Form 222, can you just cross out the error?
No. If an error is made, then all copies of the 222 form must be voided and retained in the pharmacy records.

How many carbon copies are attached to a DEA Form 222?
2 copies. In total, you have the original, plus 2 copies.

What color is each copy of a DEA Form 222?
- The first page (original) is brown.
- The second page (first carbon copy) is green.
- The third page (second carbon copy) is blue.

When ordering Schedule II drugs for your pharmacy, what do you do with the first two pages (brown and green) of the DEA Form 222?
Give them to the supplier without separating them. For the form to be valid from the supplier's perspective, the brown and green copies must be intact with the carbon paper between them.

Which part of the DEA Form 222 is the supplier required to retain?
The first page (brown copy).

Which part of the DEA Form 222 does the supplier forward to the DEA?
The second page (green copy).

Which part of the DEA Form 222 is the pharmacy required to retain?
The third page (blue copy).

How long are you required to maintain records of your 222 forms?
2 years.

What is the DEA Form 222a used for?
Ordering more DEA 222 Forms.

What is the DEA Form 106 used for?
Reporting loss or theft of controlled substances.

What is the DEA Form 104 used for?
Closing a pharmacy/surrendering a pharmacy permit.

What is the DEA Form 41 used for?
Reporting the destruction of controlled substances.

Doctor of Medicine (MD)
Doctor of Osteopathic Medicine (DO)
Doctor of Dental Medicine (DMD)
Doctor of Dental Surgery (DDS)
Doctor of Optometry (OD)
Doctor of Podiatric Medicine (DPM)
Doctor of Veterinary Medicine (DVM)
Physician Assistant (PA)
Nurse Practitioner (NP)

Do pharmacists have prescribing authority?
In some states (e.g. New Mexico, North Carolina, Montana), pharmacists can obtain the authority to initiate medication therapy. Many other states allow pharmacists to have more limited prescriptive authority. Check with your state board of pharmacy to find out what the rules are in your state.

Can dentists prescribe medications to treat depression?
No, prescribers cannot prescribe medications to treat conditions outside of their scope of practice. For instance, a DVM cannot prescribe medications for a human, a DPM cannot prescribe medications to treat conditions of the eye, and an OD cannot prescribe medications to treat conditions of the foot, etc.

Note: State law may extend prescriptive authority to other healthcare professionals (e.g. certified nurse-midwives).

Sample DEA#: MH4836726

Why and how would I determine if a prescriber's DEA number is valid?
A prescriber cannot legally issue a controlled substance prescription unless he/she has obtained a DEA registration number. That number must appear on the face of any controlled substance prescription which he/she issues. You may want to verify a DEA number before dispensing a controlled substance, especially if prescription forgery is suspected. There are two components of a DEA number: the letters and the numbers. First we will look at the letters.

The 1st Letter: DEA numbers begin with 2 letters. The 1st letter of the DEA number provides information about the type of practitioner or registrant.
- A, B, or F for physicians, dentists, veterinarians, hospitals, and pharmacies.
- M for midlevel practitioners.
- P or R for drug distributors.

Note: prescribers who have been granted a DEA waiver to write prescriptions for Subutex® or Suboxone® outside of a narcotic treatment program will have a DEA number that begins with the letter "X."

The 2nd Letter: The second letter of the DEA number will be the same as the first letter of the prescriber's last name or the first letter in the name of the business.

Now that you know what the letters in a DEA number represent, let's see how to go about verifying the numerical portion of a DEA number.

---Step 1---
Add the 1st, 3rd, and 5th digits of the DEA number.

---Step 2---
Add the 2nd, 4th, and 6th digits of the DEA number and multiply the sum by 2.

Note: Remember to multiply the correct set of numbers by 2. If you multiply the sum of the 1st, 3rd, and 5th digits by 2, you will get the wrong answer.

---Step 3---
Take your answer from "Step 1" and add it to your answer from "Step 2."

---Step 4---
Your answer for "Step 3" will be a 2 digit number. If the DEA number is valid, then the second digit of the two digit number from "Step 3" will match the 7TH and final digit of the DEA number. For example, let's say your answer from "Step 3" was 4<u>8</u>. If the DEA number was valid, then the DEA number would end with the number 8. Now try it yourself. Use this 4-step process to verify the sample DEA# shown at the top of the page.

Practice Problem
Verify the example DEA number below.

John Smith, MD
DEA # FS8524616

Solution:
- The registrant is a physician (MD), so the first letter must be "A, B, or F."
- The prescriber's last name is Smith, so the second letter must be "S."
- The sum of the 1st, 3rd, and 5th numbers (8 + 2 + 6) is 16.
- The sum of the 2nd, 4th, and 6th numbers (5 + 4 + 1) is 10, and 10 x 2 = 20.
- The sum of 16 and 20 is 3<u>6</u>.
- The last number of the DEA number is 6, which is the same as the second digit of the number 36.
- According to our analysis, this DEA number appears to be valid.

Note: The "Drug Addiction Treatment Act of 2000" (DATA 2000) is the name of the law that requires prescribers to include their special DEA number (which starts with the letter "X") on prescriptions written for Subutex® or Suboxone®.

How did the Poison Prevention Packaging Act of 1970 change the way we dispense drugs?
This act required drugs to be dispensed in child-resistant packaging. There are several exceptions; one of which is nitroglycerin sublingual tablets.

Why are nitroglycerin sublingual tablets exempt from the PPPA?
Nitroglycerin sublingual tablets are used to restore blood flow to the heart during an exacerbation of angina (characterized by acute chest pain), potentially preventing a myocardial infarction (heart attack). Child resistant packaging may cause an individual on the verge of a heart attack to struggle with opening the container of this potentially life-saving medication (nitroglycerin). As a result, this medication is exempt from the rules of the PPPA.

What is the intent of the PPPA?
The PPPA is intended to protect children from serious injury or illness caused by handling, using, or ingesting medications and certain household substances.

How is this accomplished?
The PPPA protects children by requiring manufacturers to use packaging that is *significantly difficult* for children under the age of 5 years old to open, yet not difficult for normal adults to open.

How did the Omnibus Reconciliation Act of 1990 (OBRA '90) change pharmacy practice?
By requiring drug utilization reviews (DUR) and pharmaceutical care (i.e. pharmacist counseling) for Medicaid patients.

If OBRA '90 only requires an offer for pharmacist counseling to be made to Medicaid patients, why does *every* customer (including non-Medicaid customers) receive the same offer?
The "offer to counsel" became part of standard pharmacy business practices to ensure that all customers were receiving the same level of service.

What is the purpose of the Health Insurance Portability and Accountability Act of 1996 (HIPAA)?
To protect the privacy of individual health information (referred to in the law as "protected health information" or "PHI").

If an individual's PHI has been breached, what must be done according to HIPAA?
The individual must be notified by the person or entity holding the information that their PHI was exposed. This is known as the "HIPAA Breach Notification Rule."

Does HIPAA set standards for protecting *electronic* PHI, such as electronic medical records (EMR)?
Yes.

When using or disclosing PHI, what principle should you keep in mind?
The principle of "minimum necessary use and disclosure."

To which situation(s) does the principle of "minimum necessary use and disclosure" not apply?
- Disclosures to a healthcare provider for treatment.
- Disclosures to the patient upon request.
- Disclosures authorized by the patient.
- Disclosures necessary to comply with other laws.
- Disclosures to the Dept. of Health and Human Services (HHS) for a compliance investigation, review, or enforcement.

Pseudoephedrine can only be purchased from what location?
Behind the pharmacy counter or from a locked cabinet stored away from customers.

True or false. Pseudoephedrine can be purchased without a photo ID.
False.

What packaging requirement applies to solid oral dosage forms of pseudoephedrine?
They must be packaged and sold in blister packs; pseudoephedrine can never be sold as loose tablets/capsules.

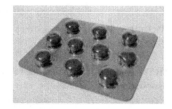

Daily sales of pseudoephedrine are limited to what amount?
3.6 grams/day.

Monthly (30-day) sales of pseudoephedrine are limited to what amount?
9 grams/30 days.

Federal law limits the amount of pseudoephedrine purchased via mail order to what amount over a 30-day period?
7.5 grams.

What information must be logged during the sale of products containing pseudoephedrine?
- Product name.
- Quantity sold.
- Name and address of purchaser.
- Date and time of sale.
- Signature of purchaser.

Records from pseudoephedrine sales must be kept for what length of time?
2 years.

What is a hazardous drug?
A hazardous drug is a medication that, upon exposure, can cause harm to human or animal life. For example, exposure to a hazardous drug may cause reproductive toxicity, organ damage, birth defects, and/or cancer.

In which drug classes do we find most hazardous drugs?
Cancer chemotherapy, antivirals, immunosuppressants, hormones, and certain anticonvulsants.

Why would a patient receive a hazardous drug?
Consider a patient with cancer. The cancer, if left untreated, could grow and spread very quickly. Now imagine that there is a drug that could slow, and potentially stop, the cancer growth, but this drug is known to cause liver toxicity. For our patient with cancer, the benefit of slowing or stopping the cancer is likely to outweigh the risk of liver toxicity.

When handling hazardous drugs, healthcare workers should follow _____ and any recommendations included in the manufacturer's _____.
- Standard precautions
- Material safety data sheet (MSDS)

What are the standard precautions that should be followed by healthcare workers when handling hazardous drugs?
- Store hazardous drugs in a well-ventilated area separate from all other inventory.
- Wear chemotherapy gloves whenever handling hazardous drugs (e.g. when receiving, stocking, counting inventory, preparing for administration, and disposing).
- Perform sterile compounding activities with hazardous drugs in an ISO class 5 biological safety cabinet or compounding aseptic containment isolator.
    - o The safety cabinet or containment isolator used for compounding hazardous drugs must be physically separated from other sterile compounding preparation areas.
- Wear appropriate personal protective equipment (PPE) when compounding products that contain hazardous drugs.
    - ▪ Gown.
    - ▪ Face mask.
    - ▪ Eye protection.*
    - ▪ Hair cover.
    - ▪ Shoe covers.
    - ▪ Double-gloving with sterile chemotherapy gloves.*

*Precautions that are not routinely recommended for compounding non-hazardous sterile drug products.

Why is it necessary for healthcare workers to follow standard precautions when handling hazardous drugs?
When healthy individuals are exposed to a hazardous medication they risk experiencing the potential adverse effects associated with using the drug, but with no therapeutic benefit.

What organizations provide information regarding the storage, handling, and disposal of hazardous drugs?
- United States Pharmacopoeia (USP)
- American Society of Health-System Pharmacists (ASHP)
- National Institute for Occupational Safety and Health (NIOSH)
- Occupational Safety and Health Administration (OSHA)

What information is provided in a product's material safety data sheet (MSDS)?
- Chemical and physical properties.
- Health, safety, fire, and environmental hazards.
- Information on what to do if the product is accidentally spilled.

The information provided in a material safety data sheet is intended to be used by _____ & _____.
- Workers that will potentially be exposed to chemicals.
- Emergency response personnel (e.g. firefighters).

Who is responsible for making MSDSs available to employees?
The employer.

What type of container must be used for the disposal of hazardous drug-contaminated needles and syringes?
Chemotherapy sharps container.

How does one distinguish a standard sharps container from a *chemotherapy* sharps container?
Standard sharps containers are red & chemotherapy sharps containers are yellow.

What is the purpose of a black pharmaceutical waste container?
Black pharmaceutical waster containers are used for the disposal of bulk hazardous drug waste (e.g. disposal of a partially empty vial of a cancer chemotherapy drug).

All areas where hazardous drugs are routinely handled must contain:
Hazardous drug spill kits, containment bags, and disposal containers.

What supplies should be included in a hazardous drug spill kit?
- Material to absorb about 1,000 mL of liquid
    - o Plastic-backed, absorbent spill cleanup pads
    - o Disposable towels
- Personal protective equipment (PPE)
    - o Two (2) pairs of gloves
    - o Gown
    - o Shoe covers
    - o Face shield
- Two (2) or more sealable plastic hazardous waste disposal bags
- One (1) disposable scooper and one (1) puncture-resistant container for collecting and disposing of broken glass.

Note: all spill cleanup materials must be disposed of as hazardous waste.

What steps should one take in the event of exposure to a hazardous drug by direct skin or eye contact?
- Call for help (if necessary).
- Remove any contaminated clothing.
- Wash affected eye(s) with water for at least 15 minutes.
- Clean affected skin with soap & water. Rinse well.
- Seek medical attention & document the exposure.

Hazardous Drugs – Select Examples

Drug Class	Generic Drug Name
Cancer chemotherapy	Anastrozole
	Bicalutimide
	Cisplatin
	Exemestane
	5-Fluorouracil
	Letrozole
	Mercaptopurine
	Methotrexate
	Oxaliplatin
	Tamoxifen
	Vinblastine
	Vincristine
Antivirals	Abacavir
	Entecavir
	Ganciclovir
	Valganciclovir
	Zidovudine
Immune system suppressants	Azathioprine
	Cyclosporine
	Mycophenolate
	Sirolimus
	Tacrolimus
Anticonvulsants	Carbamazepine
	Divalproex
	Oxcarbazepine
	Phenytoin
Hormones	Estorgens
	Progestins
	Medroxyprogesterone

All medications have benefits (the intended therapeutic effect) and risks (side effects). Some drugs have higher risks than others. Drugs with unacceptably high levels of risk typically do not reach the market or, if they have already reached the market, are withdrawn from the market (e.g. Vioxx®). What do you do when you have a medication with a very high level of risk that has a tremendous benefit for some patients? The answer is: restricted drug programs, also referred to as Risk Evaluation and Mitigation Strategies (REMS). The FDA, pursuant to the FDA Amendments Act of 2007, can require manufacturers to comply with REMS to manage the risks associated with certain drugs. REMS are meant to ensure that the benefits of using a particular medication outweigh the associated risks.

What consequence can a manufacturer face for failing to comply with REMS?
A fine of at least $250,000 per incident.

Can manufacturers implement a REMS program without being required by the FDA to do so?
Yes.

Approximately how many drugs have a REMS program?
Over 100 drugs.

What are some of the most well-known and frequently used REMS programs?
iPLEDGE™, THALIDOMID REMS™, T.I.P.S., and Clozaril® National Registry.

What is iPLEDGE™?
iPLEDGE™ is a REMS program with two primary aims: ensuring patients who begin isotretinoin therapy are not pregnant and preventing pregnancy in patients who receive isotretinoin therapy. Why? Isotretinoin has been linked to *severe birth defects* when used during pregnancy.

> Note: several brand name formulations of isotretinoin are available: Absorbica®, Accutane®, Amnesteem®, Claravis®, Myorisan®, Sotret®, and Zenatane®.

THALIDOMID REMS™ (formerly known as S.T.E.P.S. ®)
The THALIDOMID REMS™ program was previously known as S.T.E.P.S.® (System for Thalidomide Education and Prescribing Safety). Thalomid® (thalidomide) can be used for the treatment of multiple myeloma and erythema nodosum leprosum, but the drug causes *severe birth defects and venous thromboembolic events* (i.e. deep vein thrombosis and pulmonary thromboembolism) in patients who use the drug. Similar to isotretinoin, thalidomide can never be used in women who are pregnant or may become pregnant.

T.I.P.S.

Tikosyn In Pharmacy System (T.I.P.S.) is a REMS program aimed at communicating the risk of induced cardiac arrhythmia associated with the use of Tikosyn® (dofetilide). Tikosyn® (dofetilide) is used to induce and maintain normal cardiac sinus rhythm in highly symptomatic patients with atrial fibrillation or atrial flutter of more than one week. The major issue with this drug is that it can actually cause *potentially fatal ventricular arrhythmias*, especially in patients who are starting or re-starting therapy. For this reason, patients receiving this drug must be admitted to a facility for medical monitoring for at least 3 days when starting or re-starting therapy with this drug.

Clozaril® National Registry

The Clozaril® National Registry is essentially a database for recording and referencing the white blood cell count (WBC) of patients who are receiving therapy with clozapine. Clozaril® (clozapine) is used in the treatment of various psychiatric disorders (e.g. schizophrenia, bipolar disorder). The problem with clozapine is the *potentially fatal side effect of agranulocytosis* (suppression of white blood cell production). For this reason, white blood cells must be measured by a medical lab and recorded in the Clozaril® National Registry on a weekly basis for the first 6 months of therapy and periodically thereafter. Pharmacies can only dispense enough of the drug to treat the patient until their next scheduled lab work (e.g. a 7-day supply every week for the first 6 months of therapy). This program has been referred to as the "no blood, no drug" program.

Do all REMS programs require as much work as iPLEDGE™, THALIDOMID REMS™, T.I.P.S., and the Clozaril® National Registry?

No. In fact some REMS programs are so simple you might be surprised to know that they are even considered REMS programs. One example is Dulera® (mometasone furoate/formoterol). The only requirement for the Dulera® REMS program is that the increased risk of asthma-related death associated with the use of long-acting beta agonists (such as the formoterol found in Dulera®) must be communicated to healthcare professionals and prescribers.

How does a drug obtain FDA approval for use in humans?
Drugs are approved by the FDA only after they have been proven safe and effective through clinical trial data. Clinical trials are composed of four phases (see below), and the process of obtaining FDA approval usually takes several years.

Phase 1 Clinical Trials
- Small study involving 20 - 80 healthy male volunteers.
- Low doses tested.
- Data collected on drug bioavailability & dose needed to elicit a response.

Phase 2 Clinical Trials
- Study involving 40 - 300 patients with the disease of interest.
- Minimum effective dose and maximum toxic dose determined.
- Side effects experienced by the test subjects recorded.

Phase 3 Clinical Trials
- Study involving 300 – 3,000 patients of various gender, race, lifestyle, and age.
- Risks and benefits of using the drug assessed.
- Drug formulation refined.
- Placebo studies conducted.

Post-marketing Surveillance
- Information continually gathered about the safety & effectiveness of a drug after it has been approved and marketed.
- Some drugs are removed from the market due to revelations from post-marketing surveillance. For example, Vioxx® (rofecoxib) was a COX-2 inhibitor removed from the market when post-marketing surveillance revealed an increased risk of heart attack and stroke.

KNOWLEDGE DOMAIN #3
STERILE AND NON-STERILE COMPOUNDING
(8.75% OF EXAM)

What is compounding?

In a way, compounding is like manufacturing on a very small scale; however, legislators have gone to great lengths to make distinctions between compounding and manufacturing. Compounding can take place in a registered pharmacy under the supervision of a licensed pharmacist, but manufacturing cannot. Likewise, manufacturing can take place in a facility that is registered as a drug manufacturing business, but compounding cannot. So, what exactly is compounding then? Compounding is the creation of personalized, *patient-specific* medications. For instance, a patient who is unable to swallow pills may need to receive a drug that is only available commercially as an oral tablet. In cases like this, the pharmacy may be called upon to compound a customized version of the medication (e.g. an oral liquid version of the medication).

How does the law distinguish between compounding pharmacies and manufacturers?

Compounding pharmacies must adhere to these basic guidelines (among others):

- A compounded drug product cannot be a copy of a commercially available FDA-approved product.
- A compounded drug product cannot contain any ingredient that has been deemed unsafe or ineffective.
- Products can only be compounded after receiving an individual, patient-specific prescription order (or in anticipation of receiving a patient-specific prescription order where an established prescribing pattern exists).

Now that you understand what compounding is, let's take a look at some standard compounding equipment and the math you will need to use when compounding a drug product.

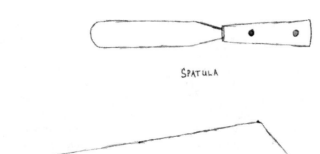

SPATULA

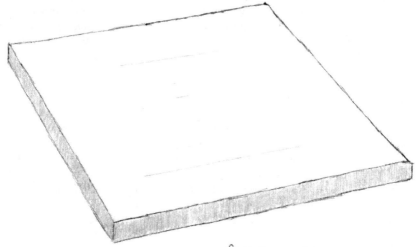

GLASS OINTMENT SLAB

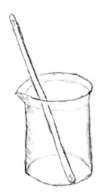

BEAKER &
GLASS STIRRING ROD

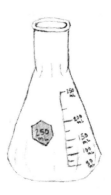

ERLENMEYER FLASK

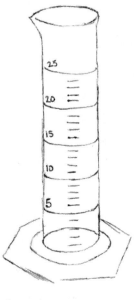

GRADUATED CYLINDER

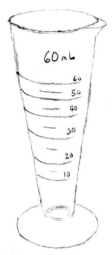

CONICAL GRADUATE

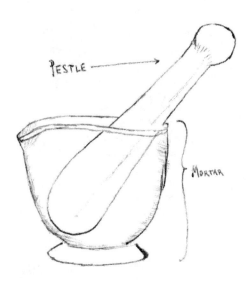

PESTLE ⟶

MORTAR

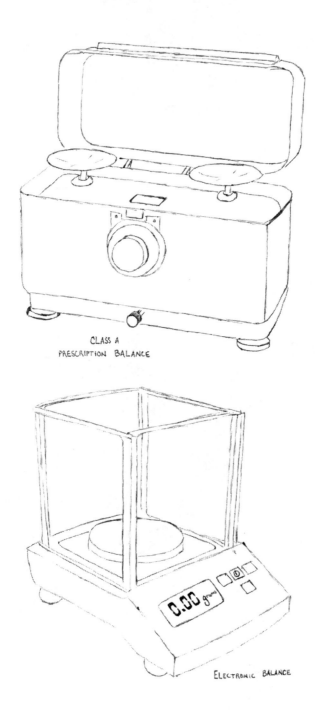

CLASS A
PRESCRIPTION BALANCE

ELECTRONIC BALANCE

Note: a class A prescription balance is the standard, traditional balance used in pharmacies for measuring the weight of ingredients when compounding medications. Most pharmacists these days use an electronic balance, which is easier to use and potentially more accurate.

Look at the image below. If each hashmark represents one milliliter, how many milliliters of gray liquid are contained in the measuring device?

    A. 32 mL
    B. 31 mL
    C. 30 mL
    D. 29 mL

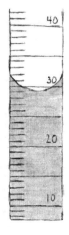

See following page for answer and explanation.

Answer: D. 29 mL

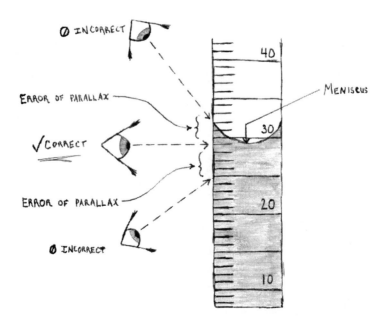

There is only one right way to measure a liquid using a liquid measuring device, and that is *at the bottom of the meniscus* (the curve at the surface of the liquid) and *at eye level*. When measurements are made above or below eye level, the difference between the actual level and the apparent level of liquid in the device is called the "error of parallax."

Weight/Weight % (w/w) = # of grams of API* per 100 grams of preparation.
   Example
   AndroGel® 1% gel contains 1 g testosterone per 100 grams of gel.

   Practice Problem
   How many milligrams of testosterone are contained in one 5-gram packet of AndroGel® 1% gel?

$$\frac{1\text{ g testosterone}}{100\text{ g gel}} \times \frac{5\text{ g gel}}{1} \times \frac{1{,}000\text{ mg}}{\text{g}} = 50\text{ mg testosterone}$$

Weight/Volume % (w/v) = # of grams of API* per 100 mL of preparation.
   Example
   Clindamycin 1% topical solution contains 1 g clindamycin per 100 mL of solution.

   Practice Problem
   What is the percent concentration (w/v) of a 250-mL solution that contains 35 mg of an active ingredient?

$$\frac{0.035\text{ g}}{250\text{ mL}} = \frac{x}{100\text{ mL}} \quad \therefore \quad x = \frac{0.035\text{ g} \times 100\text{ mL}}{250\text{ mL}} = 0.014\text{ g}$$

0.014 g/100 mL = 0.014% (w/v)

Volume/Volume % (v/v) = # of mL of API* per 100 mL of preparation.
   Example
   Charatussin® AC contains 3.8% (v/v) alcohol, meaning that it contains 3.8-mL of alcohol in every 100-mL of Cheratussin® AC solution.

   Practice Problem
   What is the percent concentration (v/v) of a 15-mL bottle of a solution that contains 0.75-mL tea tree oil in sterile water?

$$\frac{0.75\text{ mL API}}{15\text{ mL}} = \frac{x}{100\text{ mL}} \quad \therefore \quad x = \frac{0.75\text{ mL API} \times 100\text{ mL}}{15\text{ mL}} = 5\text{ mL}$$

5 mL/100 mL = 5% (v/v)

*API = active pharmaceutical ingredient

When expressing a concentration as a percent, why is it necessary to specify whether the concentration is in terms of w/w, w/v, or v/v?

It is necessary to specify because some substances can only be measured feasibly by weight (i.e. solid substances) and some substances are easier to measure by volume (i.e. liquids). Weight and volume are not equal (e.g. 1 mL of alcohol weighs 0.79 grams), except in the case of water (1 mL of water weighs 1 gram). This is because different substances have different densities (see section titled "Density and Specific Gravity" for more details on density).

More Practice Problems

1. A 6-month-old female is given one-half dropperful of Sodium Fluoride 0.11% (w/v) drops. How many milligrams of Sodium Fluoride did she receive?
Note: 1 dropperful = 1 mL

2. Clobetasol propionate topical solution comes in a 50-mL bottle. If each mL of solution contains 0.5 mg of clobetasol propionate, what is the percent concentration of the solution?

3. Prednisolone 15 mg/5 mL oral solution contains 5% (v/v) alcohol. How many milliliters of alcohol are there in one teaspoonful of solution?

4. Antipyrine and benzocaine otic solution contains 1.4% (w/v) benzocaine and 5.4% (w/v) antipyrine in an anhydrous glycerin base. How many milligrams of each active ingredient are present in one 15-mL bottle?

Practice Problem Answers
1. 0.55 mg Sodium Fluoride
2. 0.05% (w/v)
3. 0.25 mL alcohol
4. 810 mg of antipyrine & 210 mg of benzocaine

Ratios are used in:
1. Compounding recipes.
2. Expressing the concentration of a liquid medication.

Ratios Used in Compounding Recipes

When used in a compounding recipe, ratios describe how many parts of each substance make up the whole. For instance, a 24-ounce cherry pie recipe that calls for a 1:1 ratio of pie dough to cherry filling would be composed of 12 ounces of pie dough and 12 ounces of cherry filling.

An order for a compounded medication will include (at minimum) this basic information:
1. The names of each ingredient.
2. The amount or ratio of each ingredient.
3. The amount of final product desired.*

* In some cases, the amount of final product desired may be written by the prescriber as "QS," which comes from the Latin phrase "quantum sufficit" meaning "as much as suffices." In these cases, you will need to calculate how much to prepare based on the dosing instructions. See the following example.

Example Problem

What volume of each ingredient would be needed to compound the following prescription?

James Smith, D.O.
Simplified Medical Clinic • 10001 N. Main St. Suite 100A
Simple City, USA 24680
Telephone: (123) 555-1234

Name George Simpleton   Age 50
Address 2220 N. Main St. Simple City, USA 24680   Date 1-14-2015

Rx   1 Part Viscous Lidocaine : 2 Parts Diphenhydramine 12.5 mg/5 mL

Dispense QS   Elixir

Sig : Swish & Swallow 3 tsp. QID x 14 days

| NR | 1 | 2 | 3 | 4 | 5 | PRN |

James Smith   , D.O.

Prescriber Must Write "Brand Name Medically Necessary" on the Prescription to Prohibit Generic Substitution.

Solution:

Step 1: *Since the quantity is written as QS, you must calculate the amount of final product desired. This is easy, because you know how much product is being used in one dose (3 teaspoonsful), you know how many doses the patient will take each day (4 doses/day), and you know how long the patient will be taking the medication (14 days).*

$$\frac{15\,\text{mL}}{\text{dose}} \times \frac{4\,\text{doses}}{\text{day}} \times \frac{14\,\text{days}}{1} = 840\,\text{mL}$$

Step 2: *Calculate the amount that makes up 1 part of the 3 part mixture by dividing the amount of final product desired by 3 parts.*

$$\frac{840\,\text{mL}}{3\,\text{parts}} = 280\,\text{mL/part}$$

Step 3: *Now that you know the amount that represents 1 part, calculate the amount of each ingredient that will be needed to compound the prescription.*

$$\frac{1\,\text{part Lidocaine 2\%}}{1} \times \frac{280\,\text{mL}}{\text{part}} = 280\,\text{mL Lidocaine 2\%}$$

$$\frac{2\,\text{parts Diphen. 12.5mg/5mL}}{1} \times \frac{280\text{mL}}{\text{part}} = 560\,\text{mL Diphen. 12.5mg/5mL}$$

Answer: 280 mL Lidocaine 2% & 560 mL diphenhydramine 12.5 mg/5 mL

Ratios Used to Express the Concentration of a Medication

When used to express a concentration, a ratio describes how many parts of the active ingredient are present in a certain number of parts of the total formulation. For example, epinephrine 1:10,000 solution contains one part epinephrine in 10,000 parts of solution. The conversion factors below are for your reference.

Conversion Factors for Concentrations Expressed by a Ratio
1:1 = 1 gram per mL = 1 g/mL
1:1,000 = 1×10^{-3} grams per mL = 1 mg/mL
1:1,000,000 = 1×10^{-6} grams per mL = 1 mcg/mL

Example Problem
How many milligrams of epinephrine are there in 2 milliliters of Epinephrine 1:1,000,000 solution?

Solution:

Step 1: *Convert the ratio into a value with metric units using the conversion factor above.*

According to conversion factor above, 1:1,000,000 = 1 mcg/mL.

Step 2: *Apply the following equation or use the unit conversion/proportion approach.*

$$\frac{Weight_1}{Volume_1} = \frac{Weight_2}{Volume_2}$$

Insert the given information into the equation.
Weigth $_1$ = 1 mcg
Volume $_1$ = 1 mL
Weight $_2$ = ?
Volume $_2$ = 2 mL

$$\frac{1\ mcg}{1\ mL} = \frac{Weight_2}{2\ mL}$$

Step 3: *Get the unknown value (Weight₂) alone.*

$$Weight_2 = \frac{1\ mcg \times 2\ mL}{1\ mL} = 2\ mcg$$

Answer: 2 mcg

Practice Problems
1. The package for EpiPen Jr 2-Pak® comes with 2 Auto-Injectors, each one containing 0.3 mL of a 1:2000 epinephrine solution. How many milligrams of epinephrine are in one EpiPen Jr 2-Pak®?

2. What is the ratio strength of a 20-mL solution that contains 200 mcg of drug?

3. What is the ratio strength of a solution that contains 1 mg of drug per mL of solution?

4. How many milliliters of a 1:200 stock solution of Lidocaine would be required to compound a prescription for 50 mL of 0.25% Lidocaine solution?

5. If you have 1 gallon of a 1:40 solution of Drug XYZ, how many Liters of 1:1,000 solution of Drug XYZ can you compound?

Practice Problem Answers

1. 0.3 mg (0.15 mg of epinephrine per Auto-Injector, and there are two Auto-Injectors in one EpiPen Jr 2-Pak®)
2. 1:10,000
3. 1:1,000
4. 25 mL
5. 94.6 L

Alligation is a great way to solve certain compounding math problems. Use alligation when you are given two products with different concentrations of the same drug and you need a concentration that falls somewhere in the between (or when you have a higher concentration than what is desired and you want to dilute it with an inert substance like water or petrolatum). Start by drawing an X with a hollow center.

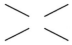

In every alligation problem, you will have to compound a prescription for a certain concentration using two products. One product will have a higher-than-desired concentration, and the other product will have a lower-than-desired concentration. For example, lets say we have a 1% cream of Product B and a 10% cream of Product B, and we want to make a cream that contains 3% Product B. Write the value for the high concentration product at the top left of the hollow X, and write the value for the low concentration product at the bottom left of the hollow X.

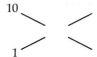

Next, write the value of the desired concentration in the center of the hollow X.

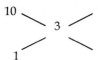

Then calculate the difference between the numbers on the left side of the X and the number at the center of the X. Write the answer, following the diagonal line, at the opposite corner of the X.

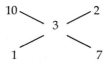

The numbers on the right side of the X indicate the proportion of each ingredient that will be needed to compound a formulation of the desired concentration.

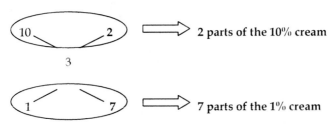

10 ⟹ 2 parts of the 10% cream

3

1 ⟹ 7 parts of the 1% cream

At this point, you would have all the information needed to solve the problem. Let's say the prescription called for 60 grams of 3% Product B cream. Based on the results of the alligation, you know that the cream would be made up of nine equal parts (2 parts of 10% cream and 7 parts of 1% cream). Divide 60 grams into nine equal parts (60 g ÷ 9 parts = 6.67 g/part). You would need 13.3 g (6.67 g/part x 2 parts = 13.3 g) of 10% cream and 46.7 g (6.67 g/part x 7 parts = 46.7 g) of 1% cream to compound 60 g of 3 % Product B cream. Now, practice as many of these as you can!

Example Problems
You need 30 g of Triamcinolone 0.05% ointment, but all you have in stock is Triamcinolone 0.025% and 0.1% ointment. How much of each ingredient will you need in order to compound this prescription?

Solution:

0.1   0.025

0.05

0.025   0.05

$$0.025 : 0.05 = 1 : 2$$

1 part 0.1% triamcinolone : 2 parts 0.025% triamcinolone

$$\frac{30 \text{ g}}{3 \text{ parts}} \times \frac{1 \text{ part } 0.1\% \text{ triamcinolone}}{1} = 10 \text{ g } 0.1\% \text{ triamcinolone}$$

$$\frac{30 \text{ g}}{3 \text{ parts}} \times \frac{2 \text{ parts } 0.025\% \text{ triamcinolone}}{1} = 20 \text{ g } 0.025\% \text{ triamcinolone}$$

Answer: 10 g of 0.1% and 20 g of 0.025% triamcinolone ointment

You have 800 mL of 70% alcohol solution. How much water will you need to add in order to make a 10% alcohol solution?
Note: Assume the water contains 0% alcohol.

Solution:

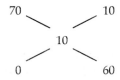

$$10 \text{ parts} = 800 \text{ mL} \therefore 1 \text{ part} = 80 \text{ mL}$$

$$60 \text{ parts} \times \frac{80 \text{ mL}}{\text{part}} = 4,800 \text{ mL}$$

Answer: 4,800 mL of water

How many grams of pure Sodium Chloride must be added to 10 mL of normal saline solution to create a 3% NaCl solution?
Note: Pure NaCl is 100% NaCl.

Solution:

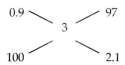

$$97 \text{ parts of } 0.9\% \text{ NaCl} = 10 \text{ mL} \therefore 1 \text{ part} = \frac{10 \text{ mL}}{97} = 0.103 \text{ mL}$$

$$2.1 \text{ parts} \times \frac{0.103 \text{ mL}}{\text{part}} = 0.22 \text{ mL} \sim 0.22 \text{ g}$$

Answer: 0.22 g of pure NaCl

You need to compound an IV solution of 2.5 mg/mL Vancomycin in D5W using a vial that contains 1 gram of Vancomycin in 20 mL. How much D5W will be needed?

Solution:

<u>Step 1</u>: *Convert the concentrations to percentages.*

> <u>Note</u>: A one-percent solution contains one gram per one hundred milliliters (1% = 1 g/100 mL). Given this fact, you can convert the given units to a percentage by calculating the number of grams in 100 mL.

$$\frac{2.5 \text{ mg}}{\text{mL}} \times \frac{\text{g}}{1{,}000 \text{ mg}} \times 100 = 0.25 \text{ g}/100 \text{ mL} = 0.25\%$$

$$\frac{1 \text{ g}}{20 \text{ mL}} \times 5 = 5 \text{ g}/100 \text{ mL} = 5\%$$

> To summarize, we are given a 5% Vancomycin solution, a 0% Vancomycin solution (D5W), and we want to create a 0.25% Vancomycin solution.

<u>Step 2</u>: *Alligation math.*

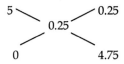

0.25 parts 5% vancomycin 4.75 parts D5W

In other words (if you multiply each part by a factor of 4), the compound must be made up of 1 part of 5% Vancomycin and 19 parts D5W.

We know we are using 20 mL of the 5% Vancomycin solution, so:

1 part = 20 mL ∴ 19 parts = 19 × 20 mL = 380 mL

Answer: 380 mL of D5W

Practice Problems
1. How much of each ingredient will be needed to make 50 mL of 1% KCl solution from 3% KCl solution and water?

2. How many Liters of 3% H_2O_2 and 6% H_2O_2 will you need to mix together to make 2 Liters of 4.5% H_2O_2?

3. You need to dilute a 5% Lidocaine cream to compound 45 grams of 4% Lidocaine cream using a cream base. How much 5% Lidocaine cream will be needed to compound this prescription?

4. How many grams of 1% Hydrocortisone cream will need to be mixed with 100% Hydrocortisone powder to make 2 ounces of 2.5% Hydrocortisone cream?
Note: 1 ounce = 28.35 grams

Practice Problem Answers
1. 16.7 mL of 3% KCl solution; 33.3 mL of water
2. 1 Liter of 3% H_2O_2 & 1 Liter of 6% H_2O_2
3. 36 grams of 5% Lidocaine cream
4. 55.8 grams of 1% Hydrocortisone cream

What does the term "aseptic" mean?
Without organisms (i.e. sterile).

What is a beyond use date (BUD)?
A beyond use date is the date after which a compounded medication should not be used. Beyond use dates are typically short (i.e. days, weeks, or months) compared to expiration dates which are usually one or more years. This is because the long-term stability of compounded medications is usually unknown.

True or false. A beyond use date and an expiration date are the same thing.
False. Manufacturers assign expiration dates to manufactured products, whereas beyond use dates are assigned to compounded drug products.

What is the technical term for a pharmacy clean room?
Buffer area.

What chapter of the United States Pharmacopoeia (USP) is concerned with compounded sterile products?
USP Chapter 797.

What is the ultimate goal of USP Chapter 797?
To protect patients from receiving contaminated infusions.

There are 5 levels of risk associated with compounded sterile products. What are the risk levels and how are they defined?

1. Immediate-use category
- Prepared using aseptic technique, but not in a clean room environment.
- Takes less than 1 hour to compound the formulation.
- Can be administered within 1 hour of compounding.
- Only for emergency situations where low-risk compounding procedures would lead to an unreasonable delay in therapy.
  - BUD 1 hour (refrigeration or room temperature)

2. Low-risk level
- Prepared using aseptic technique in a clean room environment.*
- Simple admixtures (up to 3 ingredients added with 2 entries into the infusion bag) using closed system transfer methods.
- Ingredients are sterile.
  - BUD 48 hours (room temperature)
  - BUD 14 days (refrigeration)
  - BUD 45 days (frozen at a temperature $\leq 10^{\circ}$C)

3. Low-risk level with < 12 hour BUD
- Prepared in an ISO Class 5 LAFH outside of a clean room environment (i.e. not inside a buffer area with an ante room).
- Simple admixtures (up to 3 ingredients added with 2 entries into the infusion bag) using closed system transfer methods.
- Ingredients are sterile.
- Must be administered within 12 hours of being prepared.
  - BUD 12 hours (refrigeration or room temperature)

4. Medium-risk level
- Prepared using aseptic technique in a clean room environment.
- Complex manipulations (several ingredients and entries into the bag) or extensive amount of time required to compound (e.g. TPN preparations, batch compounded preparations).
- Formulations that are to be used over several days.
- Ingredients are sterile.
  - BUD 30 hours (room temperature)
  - BUD 9 days (refrigeration)
  - BUD 45 days (frozen at a temperature $\leq 10^{\circ}$C)

5. High-risk level
- Prepared in a clean room environment.
- Ingredients are not sterile (e.g. bulk powders), or compounding method involves open system transfers.
- Improper garb.
  - BUD 24 hours (room temperature)
  - BUD 3 days (refrigeration)
  - BUD 45 days (frozen at a temperature $\leq 10^{\circ}$C)

*A *clean room environment* means in an ISO Class 5 LAFH located within an ISO Class 7 buffer area adjacent to an ISO Class 8 ante area.

The principles of sterile compounding are referred to as _____.

Highlights of aseptic technique:
⇒ Allow the laminar airflow hood to run for 30 minutes before compounding if not in continuous use.
⇒ Clean the LAFH with 70% isopropyl alcohol (wipe from top to bottom and back to front; clean all surfaces inside the hood except the screen that houses the HEPA filter).
⇒ Remove items from their packaging *before* placing them inside the hood.
⇒ Perform sterile manipulations at least 6 inches inside the outer edge of the hood (see the illustration of a laminar airflow hood below).
⇒ Do not place any objects between the HEPA filter and the sterile surfaces you that will be manipulated during compounding.
⇒ Swab surfaces with 70% isopropyl alcohol prior to puncturing (e.g. the rubber stopper on a vial; see the illustration at the top of the next page).
⇒ Do not block or disrupt the flow of air over the critical sites with your hands/fingers when manipulating the objects inside the hood (see the illustration on the bottom of the next page - notice how hand/finger positioning does not block the air flow from the LAFH).

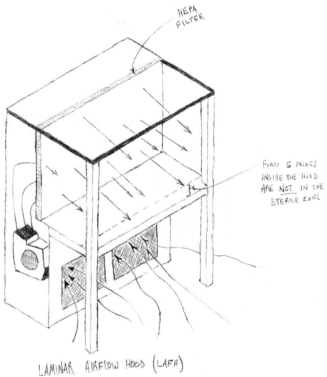

LAMINAR AIRFLOW HOOD (LAFH)

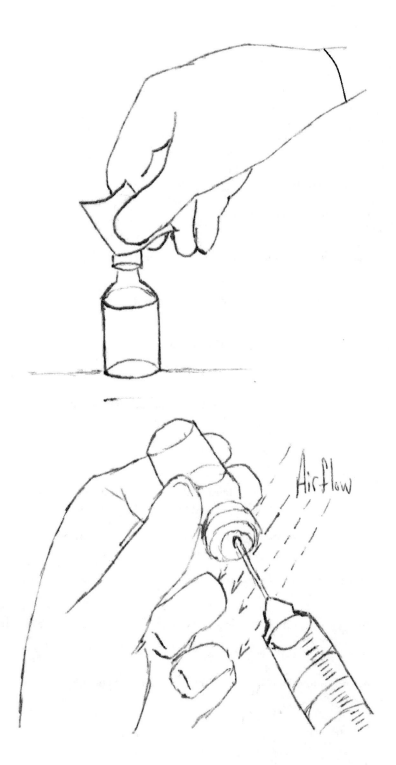

Airflow

What is a "critical site?"
The critical site is an opening that provides a pathway between the container of a sterile product and the environment. A common example of this is the rubber stopper on a vial and the needle of a syringe used to draw up the sterile liquid from the vial. When the needle punctures the rubber stopper, it creates an opening between the sterile contents of the vial and the surrounding environment.

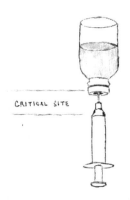

CRITICAL SITE

Sterile alcohol swabs are soaked in what type of alcohol?
70% isopropyl alcohol.

What type of container must be used for the disposal of needles?
A red sharps container.

What is the purpose of a laminar airflow hood (LAFH)?
To create an environment with a very low concentration of particles and microorganisms in the air so that formulations safe enough for human infusion can be prepared.
Note: LAFH may be abbreviated as LAFW (laminar airflow workbench).

How many air filters is a LAFH equipped with?
2 air filters (1 regular filter and 1 HEPA filter).

What is a HEPA filter?
HEPA stands for "High Efficiency Particulate Air." HEPA filters remove 99.97% of particles from the air that are 0.3 microns (micrometers) or larger.

How frequently should you wipe or spray a HEPA filter with alcohol?
Never. This would damage the filter membrane.

A LAFH must be turned on for how many minutes prior to use?
30 minutes.

Besides being turned on for 30 minutes, what else must be done prior to using a LAFH?
It must be cleaned with 70% isopropyl alcohol.

How frequently should a LAFH be cleaned with alcohol when in constant use?
Every 30 minutes.

To assure that filtered air is reaching the critical site, you must work at least __ inches inside the LAFH.
6.

In a LAFH, you want to avoid placing your hands or other objects behind the materials you are working with because you want to prevent _____.
Airflow obstruction.

What type of hood should be used to compound chemotherapy infusions?
A biological safety cabinet.

Vials have a rubber stopper. If the medication contained in a vial would undergo a chemical reaction with rubber, what type of container could the manufacturer use instead?
An ampule (an all-glass container).

Infusion filters are available with many different pore sizes. Smaller pore sizes filter out more unwanted particles, but are more prone to clogging. What are some examples of unwanted particles that filters are helpful in removing?
Glass particles, rubber fragments, dust, clothing fibers, fungi, and bacteria.

What is a micron?
A micron is a measure of length equal to one one-millionth of one meter.

What pore size is optimal for removing microorganisms, such as bacteria and fungi?
0.22 µm (referred to as a "0.22 micron filter").

What is total parenteral nutrition?
Nutrients delivered via intravenous route for the purpose of bypassing the gastrointestinal tract.

What is the difference between a TPN (total parenteral nutrition) and a TNA (total nutrient admixture)?
A TPN is a 2-in-1 mixture of amino acids and dextrose (plus electrolytes), whereas a TNA is a 3-in-1 mixture which includes the above plus a fat (lipid) component.

> Note: frequently you will hear people refer to a TNA as a TPN (as though they are synonymous), even though *technically* they are not the same type of preparation.

What would happen if you used a 0.22 micron filter on a TNA (3-in-1)?
The filter would get clogged by the fat component of the TNA.

What is the optimal pore size for filtering an infusion that contains fat (as is found in a TNA infusion)?
1.2 microns (1.2 µm).

What are the benefits and drawbacks of a 1.2 micron filter?
BENEFITS:
- Good flow of emulsified fat and other contents through the filter.
- Low probability of clogging.
- Fungi are filtered out.

DRAWBACK:
- Some bacteria and other materials smaller than 1.2 microns are not filtered out.

What is the most important compatibility consideration in TNA preparation?
The incompatibility between calcium and phosphate. If the concentration of these two ions is too high, an insoluble precipitate will form in the TNA. TNAs contain fat that turns the mixture white and opaque, making it nearly impossible to see calcium phosphate precipitates.

When compounding a TPN or TNA, how can you minimize the risk of calcium phosphate precipitate formation?
By adding phosphate toward the beginning of the compounding process and adding calcium last.

What issue must be considered when including insulin in a TPN or TNA?
Up to 50% of the insulin will bind to the surface of the inside of the bag and administration system (tubing).

What can happen when vitamin C (ascorbic acid) is included in a TPN or TNA?
Over time, ascorbic acid degrades to oxalate, which quickly binds with calcium to form an insoluble precipitate called calcium oxalate.

Why are we concerned about precipitate formation?
Precipitates are solid particles. If a solid particle is infused into a patient's bloodstream, it can get stuck in a blood vessel and block the flow of blood. This can lead to a cardiovascular event (e.g. heart attack, stroke, pulmonary embolism).

Many vials say "single-dose" on the label, indicating that the contents are preservative-free. Once the stopper of a single-dose vial is punctured, in what time frame must you to use the contents of the vial?
- If the vial is stored in less than ISO Class 5 air, you have 1 hour to use it.
- If stored in ISO Class 5 or cleaner air, you have 6 hours to use it.

True or false. Needles and syringes are sterile inside their packaging.
True.

Anatomy of a Syringe & Needle

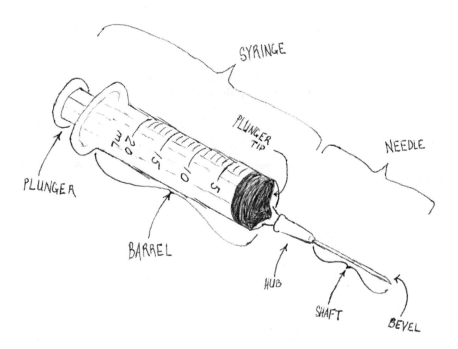

Understanding Needle Gauge Sizes

30 Gauge Needle   16 Gauge Needle

Key point: Gauge size is inversely proportional to the diameter of the needle lumen. In other words, the higher the gauge, the smaller the hole the needle creates.

Can the syringe pictured below be used to accurately measure 11 mL? Why or why not?

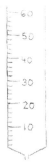

Yes. Syringes measure accurately up to one-half of the smallest marked unit. Since the syringe pictured above displays a marking for each 2 mL increment, it can be used to accurately measure to the nearest 1 mL.

When mixing medications for IV administration, it is important to look for signs of incompatibility. What are some common signs of incompatibility?
- Gas formation (bubbles)
- Precipitate formation (solid particles)
- Turbidity (cloudiness)
- Color change

Which chapter of the USP Compounding Compendium provides guidance on good compounding practices in preparing non-sterile compounded drug products?
USP Chaper 795.

What is a diluent?
A diluent is an inactive product used to dilute an active pharmaceutical ingredient.

What is trituration?
Trituration is the process of reducing the particle size of a powder, usually by use of a mortar and pestle.

What is "sensitivity requirement?"
The sensitivity requirement is the mass needed to move the balance marker by one space (see the illustration below). For a class A prescription balance, the sensitivity requirement is 6 mg.

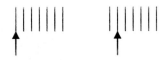

What is geometric dilution?
Geometric dilution is the process of expanding the weight of the active pharmaceutical ingredient by adding an inert substance (i.e. diluent) in a fashion that yields a homogenous mixture. In more simplified terms, you dilute the active ingredient and mix it well to ensure even mixture.

What is the purpose of geometric dilution?
Many drug doses are very small (in the microgram to milligram range). Accurately measuring these small doses can be difficult. To obtain an accurate measurement, you have two options: 1) use a highly sensitive analytical balance or 2) dilute the drug to make it weigh more. The standard pharmacy balance is a class A prescription balance. This type of balance is sensitive enough to measure 120 mg or more within 5% error. To accurately measure smaller quantities with a class A prescription balance, you must dilute the drug.

For example
If you want to measure 60 mg of a drug using a class A prescription balance, you could take 120 mg (the lowest quantity that can be accurately measured with this type of balance) of the pure (100%) drug powder and mix it with 120 mg of lactose (an inert substance; diluent). Now you have a powder that is 50% drug and 50% lactose. Now you can measure 120 mg of this mixture to obtain 60 mg of drug. The trick is to never use the balance to measure any quantity less than 120 mg. If you do, you will not stay within the 5% error requirement (to gain a better understanding of percent error, refer to the section on non-sterile compounding).

How do you perform geometric dilution?

Take the active pharmaceutical ingredient and add an equal amount of diluent. Triturate the mixture until you are convinced it is homogenous. Then add an equal amount of diluent to the mixture and triturate as before. Repeat the steps until all of the ingredients have been mixed together.

Illustrated Example of Geometric Dilution

Dilute 200 mg of amlodipine powder with 1,400 mg of lactose powder to create a homogenous mixture with a total mass of 1,600 mg.

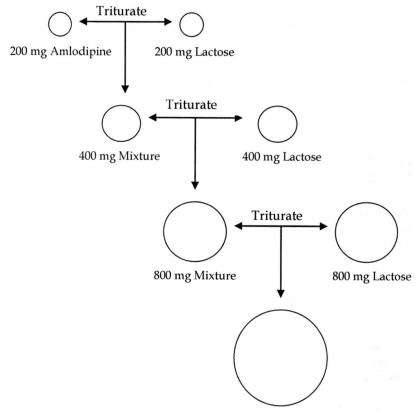

1,600 mg Mixture
(200 mg Amlodipine & 1,400 mg Lactose)

Key Point: If you just triturate 200 mg of amlodipine with 1,400 mg of lactose all in one step, you would probably achieve an uneven (heterogeneous) mixture. By slowly adding the diluent in this stepwise fashion, you greatly increase the likelihood of achieving an even (homogenous) mixture.

What is the percent error (% error)?

Percent error refers to the accuracy of a measurement. For instance, 5% error means that the measurement is within +/- 5% of the actual value. In pharmacy, the highest acceptable percent error is usually 5% but can be even less in some cases.

How are the "sensitivity requirement" and "percent error" related?

These terms are related according to the following equation:

$$\% \text{ Error} = \frac{\text{Sensitivity Requirement}}{\text{Desired Weight}} \times 100\%$$

Given that the sensitivity requirement of a class A prescription balance is 6 mg, what is the minimum quantity that can be weighed within 5% error?

Solution:

This problem can be solved using the above equation. The terms were re-written to reflect the nature of this specific question.

Note: LWQ = least weighable quantity.

$$\text{Maximum Acceptable \% Error} = \frac{\text{Sensitivity Requirement}}{\text{LWQ}} \times 100\%$$

$$5\% = \frac{6 \text{ mg}}{\text{LWQ}} \times 100\%$$

Rearrange the equation to get LWQ alone.

$$\therefore \text{ LWQ} = \frac{6 \text{ mg}}{5\%} \times 100\% = 120 \text{ mg}$$

Answer: 120 mg

If you were using a class A prescription balance to measure 20 mg of Powder X, what would the percent error be?

Solution:

$$\% \, \text{Error} = \frac{\text{Sensitivit y Requiremen t}}{\text{Desired Weight}} \times 100\% = \frac{6 \, \text{mg}}{20 \, \text{mg}} \times 100\% = 30\%$$

Answer: 30% error

Is this an acceptable level of error?
No, the highest acceptable level of error is 5%.

If you needed to measure 20 mg of a Powder X using a class A prescription balance, how would you do it while achieving a percent error ≤ 5%?
Take 120 mg of the substance (which can be measured within 5% error) and use geometric dilution to create a homogenous mixture of 1 part (120 mg) Powder X and 5 parts (600 mg) diluent (e.g. lactose). Then, using the class A prescription balance, measure out 120 mg of the mixture, which will contain 20 mg of Powder X.

You are compounding a prescription which requires you to measure 40 mL of a liquid. Which of the following pieces of equipment should you use?
  A.   10 mL graduated cylinder
  B.   50 ml graduated cylinder
  C.   20 mL syringe
  D.   60 mL syringe

Answer:
B. 50 mL graduated cylinder

Equipment Selection Tip
Use the smallest measuring device that will hold the desired volume.

Practice Problems

1. You want to measure 10 mg of a substance within 1% error without diluting it. The sensitivity requirement of your balance would need to be ___.

2. You are using a class A prescription balance to measure 9 grams of maltose. What percent error will you get with this measurement?

3. You want to measure out 20 mg of hydrocortisone within 5% error using a class A prescription balance. Since the LWQ (least weighable quantity) is 120 mg, you know you will have to perform a geometric dilution to obtain a 20 mg measurement within 5% error. How much diluent powder and hydrocortisone will need to be combined to perform the geometric dilution?

4. After completing the geometric dilution from *practice problem 3* (above), what is the ratio of hydrocortisone to diluent powder?

5. From practice problem 3, what is the percent concentration of hydrocortisone in the resulting powder mixture?

6. From practice problem 3, what is the fraction of hydrocortisone in the resulting powder mixture?

Practice Problem Answers
1) 0.1 mg
2) 0.067%
3) 600 mg of diluent powder & 120 mg of hydrocortisone
4) 1:5 hydrocortisone to diluent powder
5) 16.67%
6) 1/6

KNOWLEDGE DOMAIN #4
MEDICATION SAFETY
(12.5% OF EXAM)

Each health care organization seeking to satisfy the requirements of the National Patient Safety Goals (a set of requirements that are part of the Joint Commission accreditation* process) is responsible for developing a look-alike/sound-alike medication list. Here is an example look-alike/sound-alike list:

Aciphex and Aricept
Advair and Advicor
Alprazolam and Lorazepam
Amlodipine and Amiloride
Benadryl and Benazepril
Bupropion and Buspirone
Celebrex and Celexa**
Celebrex and Cerebyx
Clomiphene and Clomipramine
Clonidine and Klonopin**
Clozaril and Colazal
Codeine and Lodine
Diprivan and Ditropan
Dobutamine and Dopamine
Durasal and Durezol
Fioricet and Fiorinal
Flonase and Flovent
Fomepizole and Omeprazole
Glyburide and Glipizide
Guaifenesin and Guanfacene
Hydralazine and Hydroxyzine**

Kapidex and Casodex
Keppra and Keflex
Lamictal and Lamisil
Lunesta and Neulasta
Metformin and Metronidazole
Mirapex and Miralax
Misoprostol and Mifespristone
Oracea and Orencia
Oxycodone and Oxycontin
Patanol and Platinol
Pentobarbital and Phenobarbital
Prograf and Prozac
Quinine and Quinidine
Risperidone and Ropinirole
Sitagliptin and Sumatriptan
Tiagabine and Tizanidine
Tramadol and Trazadone**
Vinblastine and Vincristine**
Wellbutrin SR and Wellbutrin XL
Zantac and Zyrtec

*Joint Commission accreditation is intended to be a mark of high quality care. Health care organizations usually seek Joint Commission accreditation because, in many states, it is a precondition to receiving Medicare and Medicaid payments.
**These are some of the most problematic look-alike/sound-alike names.

1) Use tall man lettering

Tall man lettering is a way to emphasize the difference in drug names that otherwise look similar. For instance, Hydroxyzine and Hydralazine are two drug names that, at first glance, look quite similar. When you use tall man lettering, HydOXYzine and HydrALAZINE look less similar, thus reducing the chance that one will be misinterpreted as the other.

Below is a modified list from FDA.gov that demonstrates the use of tall man lettering in differentiating look-alike/sound-alike medications:

AcetaHEXAMIDE	AcetaZOLAMIDE
BuPROPion	BusPIRone
ChlorproMAZINE	ChlorproPAMIDE
ClomiPHENE	ClomiPRAMINE
CycloSPORINE	CycloSERINE
DAUNOrubicin	DOXOrubicin
DimenhyDRINATE	DiphenhydrAMINE
DOBUTamine	DOPamine
HydrALAZINE	HydrOXYzine
MethylPREDNISolone	MethylTESTOSTERone
NiCARdipine	NIFEdipine
PredniSONE	PrednisoLONE
risperiDONE	rOPINIRole
SulfADIAZINE	SulfiSOXAZOLE
TOLAZamide	TOLBUTamide
VinBLAStine	VinCRIStine

2) Separate inventory

A popular method for preventing medication dispensing errors is separating inventory. When medications are organized alphabetically, it is common to have drugs with very similar names stored right next to each another on the shelf (e.g. Isosorbide Mononitrate & Isosorbide Dinitrate or Metoprolol Tartrate & Metoprolol Succinate). The advantages of separating medications that have similar names are readily apparent. First, since the drugs are stored apart from one another, there is less of a chance that the bottles will get mixed up during storage. Second, the person filling the prescription is forced to stop and think rather than quickly reach for the first drug that appears to be correct. For instance, let's say metoprolol tartrate is stored in alphabetical order with the rest of the drugs, but the metoprolol succinate is stored on another shelf away from the rest of the inventory. When you receive an order to fill a metoprolol prescription, you remember that metoprolol is stored in two different locations. So, before you can fill the prescription, you must figure out which drug to dispense.

3) Use leading zeros

Leading zeros help to ensure accurate translation of numbers less than 1. By omitting a leading zero, you run the risk of causing the patient to receive a dose many times higher than the intended dose. This can be a fatal mistake.

Acceptable: 0.1, 0.005, 0.02, 0.99
Unacceptable: .1, .005, .02, .99

What is the difference between .99 and 0.99?
.99 could easily be misinterpreted as ninety-nine. Consider how detrimental a mistake it could be if a patient was supposed to get 0.99 grams of a drug and they ended up getting 99 grams. One hundred times the prescribed dose could cause serious adverse effects up to and including death.

4) Avoid trailing zeros

While leading zeros can prevent fatal dispensing errors, trailing zeros can cause them. Let's say a patient is prescriber issues a prescription to a patient for: Alprazolam 1 mg PO QID PRN anxiety. When writing the prescription, the prescriber uses a trailing zero, so one milligram is written as "1.0 mg." So the prescription looks like this:

Alprazolam 1.0 mg PO QID PRN anxiety

When reading this prescription, the technician and/or pharmacist might perceive the strength to be ten (10) milligrams instead of one (1) milligram. This misinterpretation could lead to a fatal dispensing error. Never use trailing zeros. Write one as 1, not 1.0 or 1.00.

5) Avoid error-prone abbreviations

Another safety strategy is avoiding the use of error-prone abbreviations. Much like leading and trailing zeros, certain abbreviations can lead to dangerous misinterpretations. The FDA and ISMP* have teamed up in a campaign to eliminate the use of error-prone abbreviations. Below is a list of some common error-prone abbreviations. As a general rule it is best to write out the instructions word for word and avoid abbreviations all together.

Error-Prone Abbreviation	Potential Misinterpretation
AD (right ear)	OD (right eye)
AS (left ear)	OS (left eye)
AU (both ears)	OU (both eyes)
OD (right eye)	AD (right ear)
OS (left eye)	AS (left ear)
OU (both eyes)	AU (both ears)
CC (cubic centimeters)	U (units)
HS (bedtime)	HS (half-strength) or HR (hour)
BT (bedtime)	BID (twice daily)
IU (international units)	IV (intravenous)
IN (intranasal)	IM (intramuscular)
QD or Q1D (daily)	QID (four times daily)
QOD (every other day)	QD (daily) or QID (four times daily)
OD (right eye)	QD (daily)
SC or SQ (subcutaneous)	5 Q ___ (five every)
ss (one-half)	55 (fifty-five)
I/d (one per day)	TID (three times daily)
º (hours; e.g. 6º = 6 hours)	0 (zero; e.g. 60 = sixty)
UD (as directed)	Unit Dose
Per Os (by mouth)	OS (left eye)

*What is the ISMP?

The Institute for Safe Medication Practices (ISMP) is a nonprofit organization that is devoted to preventing medication errors and ensuring safe use of medications.

Note: *pharmaceutical counseling* (performed by a pharmacist) is another method of reducing dispensing errors and improving safety. During pharmaceutical counseling, the pharmacist goes over important prescription information with the patient, such as the name & strength of the drug and what it is used for. This provides an excellent opportunity to recognize an error before the drug is even dispensed. For instance, let's say a patient expects to receive a prescription for tramadol (a painkiller), but during pharmaceutical counseling the patient is told by the pharmacist that the prescription that has been filled is for an antidepressant called trazodone. The patient expresses concern and explains that she was expecting a painkiller. The pharmacist retrieves the original prescription, realizes the error, and corrects the mistake immediately. Without counseling, the error could have gone unnoticed, potentially causing serious harm to the patient.

6) Read back verbal prescriptions

In certain states (assuming company policy permits), certified pharmacy technicians can accept verbal prescriptions for non-controlled substances from a prescriber (or an agent of the prescriber) over the phone. If you have this responsibility, always remember to convert the verbal order to writing immediately, write legibly, and read the order back to the prescriber (or the agent of the prescriber) to verify that all of the information was communicated correctly. This is important because, as a good friend of mine says, "What is said is not always the same as what is heard." Ignoring this safety strategy is especially dangerous when dealing with look-alike/sound-alike medications.

7) Promote patient counseling

Patient counseling is the final opportunity to catch a dispensing error before it ends up in the hands of the patient and causes harm. During a patient counseling session, the pharmacist will go over information like the brand and generic name of the medication, what the drug is used to treat, the dose prescribed, etc. Not only is this an opportunity for the patient to receive some basic education on the medicines they take, but it is also an opportunity to identify errors. For instance, let's say you drop-off a prescription for a blood pressure medication. When you go to pick up the medication, the pharmacist explains that the medication is used to treat bacterial infections and then asks you if you have an infection. You say, "No, I have high blood pressure." Disaster averted – the pharmacist realizes that this is a potential dispensing error and takes this opportunity to correct the error before it harms the patient. Even if the patient refuses counseling, try to go over the medication name with them before they purchase the medication. Make sure they know what they are receiving before they purchase the prescription.

High-alert (or high-risk) medications are drugs with a high likelihood of causing serious harm, especially when used improperly. Typically, each institution will compile a list of medications that they consider to be in the high-risk category. As a result, the medications that are considered high-risk may vary from one institution to another. Drugs from the following classes usually end up on an institution's high-alert medication list.

Anticoagulants (e.g. heparin, warfarin, enoxaparin)
These drugs are used in the treatment and prevention of blood clots, but they can cause potentially fatal *bleeding* if too much is administered to the patient.

Neuromuscular blockers (e.g. rocuronium, succinylcholine, pancuronium)
These drugs are commonly used to *stop breathing* to allow for mechanical ventilation. These drugs are usually considered to be high-risk since they take away the patient's ability to breathe.

Opioids (e.g. morphine, hydromorphone, fentanyl, meperidine)
These drugs are used to treat pain, but they can cause potentially fatal *respiratory suppression* at high doses.

Insulin (e.g. Humulin® R, Novolin® R, Humalog®, NovoLog®, Apidra®)
Insulin functions to decrease blood sugar by increasing cellular utilization of glucose in patients with diabetes, but too much insulin can cause a condition known as hypoglycemia*. In severe cases, *hypoglycemia* can be fatal.

*Hypoglycemia means low blood sugar (hypo- = low, -glyc- = sugar, -emia = blood). Symptoms of hypoglycemia include dizziness, confusion, shakiness, sweating, and heart palpitations.

Only a pharmacist can address certain situations and complete certain tasks. Some common examples are listed below.

Drug Utilization Review (DUR)
Only a pharmacist can complete a drug utilization review. The purpose of the review is to identify and respond to potential and actual drug interactions, therapeutic duplications, incorrect dosages, drug allergies, apparent drug misuse or abuse, and other medication-related issues that require professional judgment for resolution.

Therapeutic Substitution Decisions
Whenever dispensing a medication other than that originally prescribed (i.e. a generic substitute), a pharmacist must bear the responsibility of making the final decision regarding which medication to dispense.

OTC Recommendations
All requests for over-the-counter (OTC) drug recommendations must be deferred to a pharmacist.

Pharmaceutical Counseling
Anytime a patient requests counseling or has a question about a prescription drug (besides basic information such as the name and strength of the drug), pharmacist intervention is required.

Advice Regarding a Missed Dose
If a patient/customer requests advice from a technician regarding what to do in the case of a missed dose, the technician must defer to a pharmacist.

Response to an Adverse Drug Event (ADE)
A patient/customer complaining of, or asking questions about, an adverse reaction related to use of a medication should speak directly to the pharmacist.

Administration of Vaccinations/Immunizations
In a pharmacy, only a pharmacist can administer vaccinations/immunizations.

True or false. Eye drops can be used in the ear to treat conditions of the ear.
True.

True or false. Ear drops can be instilled into the eye to treat conditions of the eye.
False. Eye (ophthalmic) drops are manufactured to be bacteria-free and to contain gentle preservatives. Since the ear is not as sensitive as the eyes, ear (otic) drops are not manufactured with the same considerations as eye drops. If ear drops were administered to the eye they would cause irritation and, since ear drops are not required to be sterile, they may also cause infection.

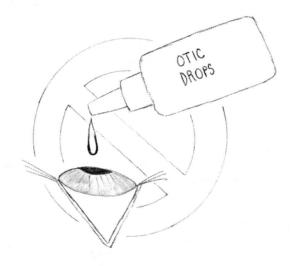

KNOWLEDGE DOMAIN #5
PHARMACY QUALITY ASSURANCE
(7.5% OF EXAM)

Bar-code technology
Use of bar-code technology has been proven to help assure quality by significantly reducing the rate of dispensing errors. Bar-code technology can be implemented during various steps of the filling and dispensing process, but the most common and impactful step where this technology can be applied is scanning the bar-code of the stock bottle after selecting the drug off of the shelf to verify the drug is correct prior to filling the prescription. Some institutions also use this technology to reduce nursing errors in medication administration (known as Bar-Code Medication Administration or "BCMA").

Matching NDC
It is important for technicians and pharmacists to ensure that the NDC number of the drug used to fill the prescription is the same as the NDC number being used to bill the insurance. It is also important when filling a prescription from more than one stock bottle of medication to ensure that all stock bottles used to fill the prescription have matching NDC numbers. Not only does this help to ensure that the patient is receiving the correct medication, but also that the insurance is being billed for the same exact product as that which is being dispensed.

Computerized physician order entry (CPOE)
Prescribers issue medication orders* by sending them electronically directly to the pharmacy department of the healthcare facility. CPOE helps to prevent errors that might otherwise occur as a result of a pharmacist misinterpreting a prescriber's handwriting.

E-prescribing
Prescribers issue prescriptions* by sending them electronically directly to the patients' pharmacy of choice. Just like CPOE, e-prescribing helps to reduce errors that might occur from misinterpretation of a prescriber's handwriting by pharmacy personnel.

*Medication orders and prescriptions are similar, yet different. A medication order is issued by a prescriber for a patient to have a drug *administered within a healthcare facility* (e.g. a hospital). On the other hand, a prescription is issued by a prescriber for a patient to receive a medication *for use outside of a healthcare facility.*

Note: some of the information from the "Sterile Compounding" section is also applicable to this section and vice versa.

What chapter of the United States Pharmacopoeia (USP) is concerned with compounded sterile products?
USP Chapter 797.

What is the ultimate goal of USP Chapter 797?
To protect patients from receiving contaminated infusions.

Personal Protective Equipment (PPE)
When compounding sterile products, it is important to follow USP Chapter 797 guidelines to assure the quality of the final product and prevent contamination by bacteria, fungi, viruses, particulate matter, etc. Next to thorough handwashing, one of the most important steps a pharmacy technician can take to reduce the likelihood of contaminating sterile products is to wear the appropriate personal protective equipment (PPE or "garb") at all times when in the clean room.

Appropriate PPE includes:
- Gown
- Shoe Covers
- Face Mask
- Beard Cover (if applicable)
- Hair Cover
- Gloves

What does it mean to "don" something?
To "don" means to put something on (e.g. to put on an article of clothing).

What is the proper order of donning PPE (also known as "garbing")?
1. Shoe Covers
2. Hair Cover
3. Beard Cover (if applicable)
4. Face Mask
****Handwashing****
5. Gown
6. Gloves

When should PPE be removed?
Only after exiting the clean room.

What is the most common cause of contamination?
Touch contamination (i.e. contact with the hand contaminates the sterile product).

When washing your hands prior to preparing a compounded sterile product (CSP), what should you use?
A. Antibacterial soap and hot water.
B. Antibacterial soap and warm water.
C. Antibacterial soap and cold water.

Answer:
B. Antibacterial soap and warm water.

What is the proper procedure for hand washing prior to entering the clean room?
Wash the hands and arms all the way up to the elbows vigorously for at least 30 seconds paying special attention to the fingernails and the spaces between the fingers.

According to USP Chapter 797, what cosmetics and accessories cannot be worn in the buffer area?
- Makeup
- Jewelry
- Watches
- Nail polish
- Artificial nails

Does USP Chapter 797 permit eating and/or drinking in the buffer area?
No.

When working with syringes and needles (e.g. when preparing sterile compounded products), why is it important to avoid recapping the needle?
Recapping a needle means that you are replacing the protective cap over the needle after it has been used. This is a dangerous practice that commonly leads to injury (people inadvertently jab themselves; this is known as a needle stick injury). Recapping is not only dangerous, but unnecessary. Red sharps containers are designed for the disposal of uncapped needles and syringes.

Class I Recalls

A recall is categorized as class I if there is a reasonable probability that use of (or exposure to) the recalled product will cause *serious adverse health consequences up to and including death.*

Class II Recalls

A recall is categorized as class II if there is a possibility that use of (or exposure to) the recalled product could cause *temporary or medically reversible adverse health consequences.*

Class III Recalls

A recall is categorized as class III if use of the recalled product is *unlikely to cause adverse health consequences.*

Review Question:
What is the most serious class of FDA recall?
Class I recall.

KNOWLEDGE DOMAIN #6
MEDICATION ORDER ENTRY AND FILL PROCESS
(17.5% OF EXAM)

"Sig" is short for the Latin term "signa," which means "to label." On a prescription, the sig is used by the prescriber to communicate the directions for use to the pharmacy. The pharmacy interprets the sig into plain English and places it on the label of the container that will be dispensed to the patient. In most cases, the sig on a prescription (i.e. the directions for use) will be written by the prescriber in abbreviated codes. An example would be: take 1 tab PO BID UD, which is translated by the pharmacy to "take one tablet by mouth twice a day as directed." Many of these abbreviations are derived from Latin or Greek words. For example, BID is an abbreviation for "bis in die," which is Latin for "twice a day." A typical sig will be composed of the following parts:

#1 – an action word
(e.g. take, give, instill, apply, place, insert, inject)

#2 – a quantity with units
(e.g. 1 tablet, 2 teaspoonsful, 4 drops, 1 gram, 1 patch, 1 suppository, 1 milliliter)

#3 – a route of administration
(e.g. by mouth, into the left eye, topically to the affected area, to the skin, rectally, vaginally, subcutaneously, intramuscularly, into each nostril, under the tongue)

#4 – the dosing frequency
(e.g. once daily, twice daily, three times daily, four times daily, every 2 hours, every 4 hours, every 6 hours, every 8 hours, every 12 hours, every other day, once a week, once a month)

See the following page for an illustration of a typical prescription.
Pay special attention to the sig.

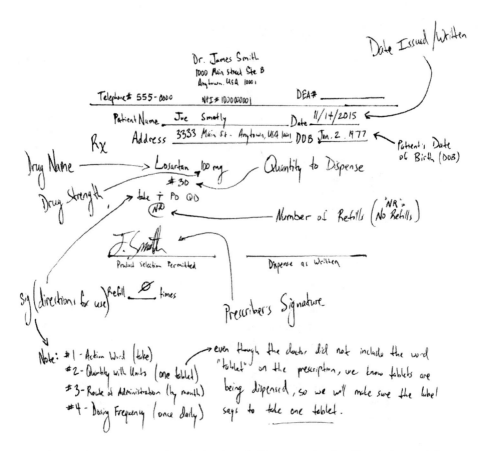

Date Issued /Written

Dr. James Smith
1000 Main street Ste B
Anytown. USA 1000 1

Telephone# 555-0000   NPI# 1000000001   DEA# _____

Patient Name ___Joe Smothly___ Date _11/14/2015_ ←

Rx   Address _3333 Main St - Anytown, USA 1001_ DOB _Jan. 2. 1977_ ←

Patient's Date
of Birth (DOB)

Drug Name ————→ Losartan 100 mg ——— Quantity to Dispense
                  # 30 ←

Drug Strength ————→ take ⊤ PO QD
                    (NR) ← ——— Number of Refills (NR = No Refills)

J. Smith ←
Product Selection Permitted   Dispense as Written

Sig (directions for use) Refill _∅_ times   Prescriber's Signature

Note: #1 - Action Word (take)   → even though the doctor did not include the word
      #2 - Quantity with Units (one tablet)   "tablet" on the prescription, we know tablets are
      #3 - Route of Administration (by mouth) being dispensed, so we will make sure the label
      #4 - Dosing Frequency (once daily)   says to take one tablet.

*Now that you know what a sig is and what it looks like, memorize the abbreviations and do
the practice problems on the following pages to gain the knowledge and experience needed to
translate sig codes competently.*

Dosing Frequency

QOD = every other day
QD = every day (daily)
BID = twice daily
TID = three times daily
QID = four times daily
QAM = every morning
QPM = every evening
Qwk = every week
Qmo = every month
H = hours
D = days
SID = once daily (used only by veterinarians)

º = hours (e.g. Q6º = every 6 hours)
hs = bedtime
ac = before meals
cf = with food
wf = with food
pc = after meals
WA = while awake
ATC = around the clock
NTE = not to exceed
PRN = as needed
STAT = immediately

Routes of Administration

PO = by mouth
PR = rectally
PV = vaginally
AU = both ears
AS = left ear
AD = right ear
OU = both eyes
OS = left eye
OD = right eye
IV = intravenous
IVP = intravenous push

IVPB = intravenous piggyback
IM = intramuscular
ID = intradermal
IC = intracardiac
IP = intraperitoneal
IN = intranasal
NG = nasogastric
SQ = subcutaneous
SL = sublingual (under the tongue)
TD = transdermal (across the skin)

Dosing Instructions

UD = as directed

AAA = apply to affected area

Dispensing Instructions

QS = sufficient quantity
NR = no refills
DAW = dispense as written (dispense brand only)

Compounding Instructions

aa = of each
ad = to make; up to
div = divide
qs ad = sufficient quantity to make

Symptoms and Disease States

N/V = nausea and vomiting
HBP = high blood pressure
HTN = hypertension
BPH = benign prostatic hyperplasia (enlarged prostate)
GAD = generalized anxiety disorder
SAD = seasonal effective disorder

Units of Measure

kg = kilogram (one thousand grams)
g = gram
mg = milligram (one one-thousandth of a gram)
μg = microgram (one one-millionth of a gram)
gr = grain (1 grain = 64.8 mg)
gtt = drop
gtts = drops
tsp = teaspoon (5 mL)
tbs = tablespoon (15 mL)
oz = ounce (one fluid ounce = 29.67 mL; one ounce of weight = 28.35 grams)
L = liter
mL = milliliter (one one-thousandth of a liter)
μL = microliter (one one-millionth of a liter)
M = molar
mM = millimolar
mEq = milliequivalent
IU = international unit

Formulations

cr = cream
crm = cream
oint = ointment
ung = ointment
lot = lotion
top = topical
inj = injection
tab = tablet
cap = capsule

susp = suspension
syr = syrup
supp = suppository
CR = controlled release
DR = delayed release
ER = extended release
LA = long acting
SR = sustained release
XR = entended release

Clean Room

PPE = personal protective equipment
D5W = 5% dextrose in water
D10W = 10% dextrose in water
NSS = normal saline solution = 0.9% sodium chloride in water
½ NS = one-half normal saline = 0.45% sodium chloride in water
D5NS = 5% dextrose in normal saline
RL = Ringer's Lactate
LR = Lactated Ringers
SWFI = sterile water for injection
LVP = large volume parenteral (infusion volume greater than 100 mL)
SVP = small volume parenteral (infusion volume equal to or less than 100 mL)
MVI = multivitamin
TPN = total parenteral nutrition

Miscellaneous

USP = United States Pharmacopoeia
NPO = nothing by mouth
D/C = discontinue
c̄ = with
s̄ = without
s̄s̄ = one-half

NKA = no known allergies
NKDA = no known drug allergies
BP = blood pressure
IOP = intraocular pressure
HRT = hormone replacement therapy

Elements/Lab Values

Ca = calcium
Cl = chloride
Fe = iron
K = potassium

Mg = magnesium
Na = sodium
Phos = phosphate
Li = lithium

Practice Problems

1. Give s̄s̄ tsp PO c̄f QID x 10D

2. Inj 12 units SQ QHS

3. Insert 1 supp PR Q6H PRN

4. 1 – 2 tabs PO Q4-6H PRN severe pain

5. 1 cap PO up to Q6H PRN N/V

6. AAA on face QPM HS

7. 1 tab PO QD for HTN

8. Inj 0.25 cc IM Qmo UD

9. Instill 1 gtt OS Q2H WA

Practice Problem Answers

1. Give one-half teaspoonful (2.5 mL) by mouth with food 4 times daily for 10 days.
2. Inject 12 units subcutaneously every night at bedtime.
3. Insert one suppository rectally every 6 hours as needed.
4. Take one to two tablets by mouth every 4 to 6 hours as needed for severe pain.
5. Take one capsule by mouth up to every 6 hours as needed for nausea and vomiting.
6. Apply to affected area on face every evening at bedtime.
7. Take one tablet by mouth once daily for hypertension.
8. Inject one-fourth mL (0.25 cc) intramuscularly every month as directed.
9. Instill one drop into left eye every two hours while awake.

APAP = Acetaminophen
ASA = Aspirin
CPZ = Chlorpromazine
DM = Dextromethorphan
EES = Erythromycin Ethylsuccinate
EPO = Erythropoietin
HC = Hydrocortisone
HCTZ = Hydrochlorothiazide
INH = Isoniazid
KCl = Potassium chloride
MgSO4 = Magnesium sulfate
MMI = Methimazole

MOM = Milk of Magnesia
MSO4 = Morphine sulfate
MTX = Methotrexate
NTG = Nitroglycerin
OC = Oral Contraceptive
PB = Phenobarbital
PCN = Penicillin
PE = Phenylephrine
PSE = Pseudoephedrine
PTU = Propylthiouracil
TAC = Triamcinolone
TCN = Tetracycline

Note: Though many prescribers still use these abbreviations, it is generally best to avoid using them due to potential misinterpretation.

There are three systems of measurement used in pharmacy. They are:

1. The apothecaries' system
2. The avoirdupois system
3. The metric system

The Apothecaries' System

Used in ancient Greece, the apothecaries' system is for the most part outdated, but a few older drugs do still have their strengths expressed in units of grains. Examples include: aspirin, ferrous sulfate, Armour Thyroid, nitroglycerin, and phenobarbital. In this system, the grain is the smallest unit of weight, and the minim is the smallest unit of volume.

Weight
1 grain (gr) = 64.8 milligrams
1 scruple (Э) = 20 grains
1 dram (ʒ) = 3 scruples
1 ounce (℥) = 8 drams
1 pound = 12 ounces

Volume
1 minim (♏) ~ 0.0617 mL
1 fluid dram = 60 minims
1 fluid ounce = 8 fluid drams
1 pint = 16 fluid ounces
1 quart = 2 pints
1 gallon = 4 quarts

The Avoirdupois System

The avoirdupois measurement system is the customary system of weights and measures in the United States. In this system, one pound equals 16 ounces.

Weight
1 grain = 64.8 mg
1 ounce (oz) = 437.5 grains
1 pound lb) = 16 ounces

Volume
1 fluid ounce = 29.57 mL
1 cup = 8 fluid ounces
1 pint = 2 cups
1 quart = 2 pints
1 gallon = 4 quarts

The Metric System

The metric system is the standard measurement system for pharmacy and medicine. As a base ten system, it is also the simplest measurement system.

Weight
1 milligram (mg) = 1,000 micrograms
1 gram (g) = 1,000 milligrams
1 kilogram (kg) = 1,000 grams

Volume
1 milliliter (mL) = 1 cm^3 (cc)
1 liter (L) = 1,000 milliliters
1 deciliter (dL) = 100 milliliters

Roman Numerals
I = 1
V = 5
X = 10
L = 50
C = 100
D = 500
M = 1,000

Rules
1) When Roman numerals are repeated, add them together.
   - Example: III = I + I + I = 3
2) When a smaller Roman numeral is written to the right of a larger Roman numeral, add it to the larger Roman numeral.
   - Example: VI = V + I = 6
3) When a smaller Roman numeral is written to the left of a larger Roman numeral, subtract it from the larger Roman numeral.
   - Example IX = X - I = 9
4) Do not use more than three of the same Roman numeral in a sequence.
   - Example: IIII = 4   IV = 4
5) When rule 2 and 3 are in conflict, use rule 3.
   - Example: XIX = 21   XIX = 19

Examples

Roman numeral III = 3
Roman numeral IV = 4
Roman numeral XIX = 19

Practice Problems
Convert the following numbers to Roman numerals:
1. 120
2. 80
3. 30
4. 3750
5. 1200
6. 473
7. 15
8. 291

Convert the following Roman numerals to numbers:

9. CL
10. XC
11. LXV
12. XLVIII
13. MM
14. CCXL
15. CDLXXX
16. CCLVI

Practice Problem Answers

1. CXX
2. LXXX
3. XXX
4. MMMDCCL
5. MCC
6. CDLXXIII
7. XV
8. CCXCI
9. 150
10. 90
11. 65
12. 48
13. 2000
14. 240
15. 480
16. 256

There are three ways to express an average: Mean, Median, and Mode.

Mean – Add up all the values and divide by the number of values.
Example
Seven values are given: 1, 4, 6, 3, 9, 8, 3
Add the seven values: $1 + 4 + 6 + 3 + 9 + 8 + 3 = 34$
Divide by seven: $34 \div 7 = 4.9$
Mean = 4.9

Median – Identify the middle value.
Example
Nine values are given: 11, 3, 10, 5, 4, 5, 5, 8, 7
Rearrange values into chronological order: 3, 4, 5, 5, 7, 8, 10, 11
Determine the middle number: 3, 4, 5, 5, **5**, 7, 8, 10, 11
Median = 5

Mode – Identify the value that appears most often in a set of values.
Example
Eight values are given: 4, 6, 7, 1, 3, 1, 3, 1
Tally the number of times each value is presented and identify the most commonly presented value:
1: III
3: II
4: I
6: I
7: I
Mode = 1

Example Problem
A patient measured her blood glucose level daily for one week. Based on her measurements, what was her mean blood glucose for the week?

Monday: 190 mg/dL
Tuesday: 182 mg/dL
Wednesday: 110 mg/dL
Thursday: 90 mg/dL
Friday: 125 mg/dL
Saturday: 130 mg/dL
Sunday: 70 mg/dL

Solution:
$$\frac{\left(190 + 182 + 110 + 90 + 125 + 130 + 70\right) \text{mg/dL}}{7} = 128 \text{ mg/dL}$$

Answer: 128 mg/dL

Practice Problems

1. What is the median in the following set of numbers: 19, 12, 49, 34, 101, 67, 1?

2. What is the mode in the following set of numbers: 4, 2, 1, 4, 5, 2, 4, 3, 2, 1, 2, 4, 2?

3. What is the mean in the following set of numbers: 3, 1, 4, 5, 2, 3, 5, 1, 5, 3, 2, 2, 4?

Practice Problem Answers
1. 34
2. 2
3. 3.1

The secret is simple – unit conversion. Many text books try to teach a more complex version of this concept that is unnecessarily difficult. The approach I am about to teach you is the same one that I successfully use to solve nearly *all* of the problems I encounter in my everyday work. The best advice to mastering this approach is to work through a lot of examples and practice problems (plenty of which you will find on the following pages). You will see this problem-solving approach applied throughout this study guide. First, *memorize* the **Must-Know Conversion Factors** (listed below) and the **Common Pharmacy Math Equations** (listed in *Appendix A* in the back of the book). Then, move on to the next page and begin solving real-world pharmacy problems! Below is the general equation you will use:

$$(\text{\# in Given Units}) \times (\text{Conversion Factor*}) = \text{\# in Desired Units}$$

*Conversion Factor = Desired Units/Given Units

Must-Know Conversion Factors

1 ounce (weight) = 28.35 g
1 fluid ounce (volume) = 29.57 mL*
Most pharmacists round up to 30 mL

1 teaspoon (tsp) = 5 mL
1 tablespoon (tbs) = 3 teaspoons = 15 mL

1 Cup = 8 fluid ounces
1 Pint = 2 cups = 16 fluid ounces
1 Quart = 2 pints = 4 cups = 32 fluid ounces
1 Gallon = 8 pints = 4 quarts = 128 fluid ounces

1 grain (gr) = 64.8 milligrams

1 gram (g) = 1,000 milligrams
1 milligram (mg) = 1,000 micrograms

1 kilogram (kg) = 2.2 pounds
1 pound (lb) = 454 grams

1 inch (in) = 2.54 centimeters

Solving pharmacy math problems is all about knowing what you are given, what you know, and where to go.

1) What you are given:
   The information provided in the problem/question.
2) What you know:
   The **Must-Know Conversion Factors** and the **Common Pharmacy Math Equations**.
3) Where to go:
   What to do with the information now that you have collected it.

Example:

A 5 year-old child has a cardiac arrhythmia. To treat the arrhythmia, the doctor prescribes propranolol at the daily dose of 0.5 mg/kg. If we determine that the child weighs 55 pounds, how many milligrams of propranolol should the child receive each day?

What you are given:
Age = 5 years old
Dose = 0.5 mg/kg
Weight = 55 lb

What you know:
Must-Know Conversion Factors
Common Pharmacy Math Equations

Where to go:
Using what you are given and what you know, you must determine how many milligrams of the medication the patient should receive each day. Everything you need to solve the problem will come from what you are given and/or what you know. All you have to do is take this information and make the units change and/or cancel out until you get the desired units.

The dose is already given in the question as 0.5 mg/kg. Now, just find a way to get the kilogram units to cancel out, and then you will have the dose in milligrams.

$$\frac{0.5\,\text{mg}}{\text{kg}} \times \frac{?}{?} \times \frac{?}{?} \ldots = ?\,\text{mg}$$

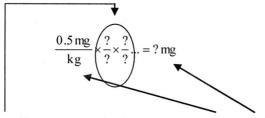

What factor(s) must you multiply by to get from here to here?

Now is the time to look back at "what you are given" and "what you know" to pick out the factors you will be able to use to cancel out the kilogram units and obtain your answer in milligrams.

What you are given:
~~Age = 5 years old~~ (age is irrelevant, because the dose is based on weight)

Dose = 0.5 mg/kg

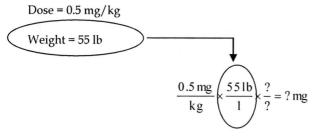

You are given the child's weight in the question. If only the weight was in units of kilograms, then you would be able to solve the problem.

What you know:

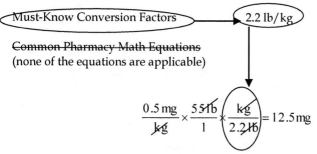

Correct Answer: 12.5 mg

The key to solving this problem was taking what you were given, combining it with what you know, and then figuring out what information/which pieces of information was/were relevant for obtaining the desired units.

Example Problems
How many fluid ounces (℥) are in 118 mL (please answer in Roman numerals)?

Solution:

> Think of the dividing line as the word "per"

$$\# \text{ in DesiredUnits} = \frac{118\,\text{mL}}{1} \times \frac{1\,\text{fluid ounce}}{29.57\,\text{mL}} = 4\,\text{fluid ounces}$$

Note: notice how the milliliter units cancel out.

Answer: IV ℥   (4 fluid ounces)

***There are 29.57 milliliters **per** fluid ounce (29.57 mL/fluid ounce). This can be written as "29.57 mL/1 fluid ounce" or "1 fluid ounce/29.57 mL." Since 1 fluid ounce is *equal* to 29.57 mL, then 29.57 mL ÷ 1 fluid ounce = 1.

Multiplying a value by the factor "29.57 mL/1 fluid ounce" is like multiplying it by 1. The actual value doesn't change, but the units do change. This is true when you multiply any number by a conversion factor.

Since multiplying by the factor "29.57 mL/1 fluid ounce" is mathematically the same as multiplying by 1, multiplying the reciprocal "1 fluid ounce/29.57 mL" is also like multiplying by 1. How do you know which way to orient the conversion factor? You have to decide which units you want on top (the numerator) and which units you want on the bottom (the denominator) based on what units you are trying to obtain. The units you are trying to obtain should go in the numerator and the units you are trying to eliminate should go in the denominator. See below for an example of what happens when you orient the conversion factor *the wrong way*:

$$\frac{118\,\text{mL}}{1} \times \frac{29.57\,\text{mL}}{1\,\text{fluid ounce}} = 3{,}489.26\,\text{mL}^2/\text{fluid ounce}$$

Clearly this did **not** give us the units we desired.

How many kilograms (kg) does a 77 lb patient weigh?

Solution:

$$\# \text{ in DesiredUnits} = \frac{77\,\text{lb}}{1} \times \frac{1\,\text{kg}}{2.2\,\text{lb}} = 35\,\text{kg}$$

Answer: 35 kg

How many milliliters are in 16 ounces?

Solution:

$$\# \text{ in Desired Units} = 16 \text{ ounces} \times \frac{29.57 \text{ mL}}{\text{ounce}} = 473 \text{ mL}$$

Note: Milliliters (mL) are the Desired Units because the question asks for an answer in milliliters. Likewise, the # in Given Units is 16 ounces, as that is the value we are given. Since we know the conversion factor (29.57 mL per ounce), we have all the information needed to solve the problem.

Answer: 473 mL

A patient drops off a prescription for 30 tablets of 5 grain ferrous sulfate. You only have four iron products stocked in the pharmacy. Which of the four products should you dispense?

    A. Fergon® (Ferrous gluconate 250 mg)
    B. Ferro-Sequels® (Ferrous fumarate 150 mg)
    C. Feosol® (Ferrous sulfate 325 mg)
    D. SlowFe® (Ferrous sulfate 225 mg)

Solution:

$$\# \text{ in Desired Units} = \frac{5 \text{ grains}}{1} \times \frac{64.8 \text{ mg}}{\text{grain}} = 324 \text{ mg}$$

Answer: C. Feosol® (Ferrous sulfate 325 mg)
Note: the answer we calculated was 1 mg lower than the answer we selected. Why is this alright? Many times, the value of 1 grain is rounded up to 65 mg. If you were to use 1 grain = 65 mg as the conversion factor (rather than 1 grain = 64.8 mg), your answer would be 325 mg. Either strength is acceptable.

You receive a prescription order for Nitrostat® sublingual tablets 1/200 grain. Nitrostat® sublingual tablets are available in 3 strengths. Which strength should you dispense?

    A. 0.3 mg
    B. 0.4 mg
    C. 0.6 mg

Solution:

$$\# \text{ in Desired Units} = \frac{1 \text{ grain}}{200} \times \frac{64.8 \text{ mg}}{\text{grain}} = 0.3 \text{ mg}$$

Answer: A. 0.3 mg

An order comes to the pharmacy for levothyroxine 0.125 mg IV injection. Using a levothyroxine 40 mcg/mL solution, how many milliliters should you dispense?
   A.   0.0031 mL
   B.   3.1 mL
   C.   0.31 mL
   D.   3.1 µL

Solution:

$$\# \text{ in Desired Units} = \frac{0.125 \text{ mg}}{1} \times \frac{1{,}000 \text{ µg}}{\text{mg}} \times \frac{\text{mL}}{40 \text{ µg}} = 3.1 \text{ mL}$$

Answer: B. 3.1 mL

A patient weighs 100.1 kg. What is the patient's weight in pounds?

Solution:

$$\# \text{ in Desired Units} = \frac{100.1 \text{ kg}}{1} \times \frac{2.2 \text{ lb}}{1 \text{ kg}} = 220 \text{ lb}$$

Answer: 220 lb

The Glucagon Emergency Kit for Low Blood Sugar, manufactured by Lilly, comes with a vial containing 1 mg of glucagon and 49 mg of lactose. Assuming Lilly has all the glucagon it needs, how many vials can they prepare using only one pound of lactose?

$$\frac{1 \text{ pound lactose}}{1} \times \frac{16 \text{ oz}}{\text{pound}} \times \frac{28.35 \text{ g}}{\text{oz}} \times \frac{1{,}000 \text{ mg}}{\text{g}} = 453{,}600 \text{ mg lactose}$$

$$\frac{453{,}600 \text{ mg lactose}}{1} \times \frac{\text{vial}}{49 \text{ mg lactose}} = 9{,}257.14 \text{ vials}$$

Answer: 9,257 vials

Sometimes the conversion factor will be given to you in the question. Take this problem for example:

What is the days' supply of a bottle of 90 tablets of levothyroxine 112 mcg if the instructions are to take one tablet by mouth every day, except take one-half tablet on Sundays?

Solution:

$$\frac{90 \text{ tablets}}{1} \times \frac{7 \text{ days}}{6.5 \text{ tablets}} = 96.9 \text{ days} \therefore 97 \text{ days}$$

Note: The conversion factor here was 6.5 tablets/7 days.

Answer: 97 days

Given a solution that contains 100 mg of drug per 5 mL, how many milliliters would be required to obtain a dose of 650 mg?

Solution:

$$\frac{650 \text{ mg}}{1} \times \frac{5 \text{ mL}}{100 \text{ mg}} = 32.5 \text{ mL}$$

Answer: 32.5 mL

Sometimes, you will need to do a series of conversions to reach the answer you need. Take this problem for example: How many 75 mcg tablets can be made from six pounds of a drug?

Solution:

$$\frac{6 \text{ pounds}}{1} \times \frac{16 \text{ ounce}}{\text{pound}} \times \frac{28.35 \text{ g}}{\text{ounce}} \times \frac{1,000,000 \text{ mcg}}{\text{g}} \times \frac{\text{tablet}}{75 \text{ mcg}}$$

= 36,288,000 tablets

Answer: 36,288,000 tablets

Practice Problems

1. How many fluid ounces are in a jug containing 3,785 mL of polyethylene glycol with electrolytes?

2. After reconstitution, how many teaspoons are in three 100-mL bottles of Amoxicillin 250 mg/5 mL oral suspension? Express your answer in Roman numerals.

3. Approximately how many tablespoons are in a 4 oz bottle of cough syrup?

4. How many scruples of aspirin are in sixteen 5 grain tablets of Ecotrin®?

5. If a patient is 6 feet tall, how tall would the patient be in centimeters?

6. You have 7 pounds of triamcinolone 0.1% ointment. How many kilograms do you have?

7. How many tablespoons are in a 150-mL bottle of an antibiotic suspension?

8. How many milliliters of a 200 mg/mL solution of testosterone cypionate should be injected intramuscularly if the patient needs to receive 75 mg per injection?

9. How many milliliters are needed to provide one 300 mg dose of amoxicillin using a 250 mg/5 mL amoxicillin suspension?

10. If a patient applies 4 g of Voltaren® 1% Gel (10 mg diclofenac/1 g gel) to her knee every day then how many milligrams of diclofenac are being applied daily?

11. A physician wrote a prescription for testosterone cypionate 200 mg/mL solution with the instructions to inject 0.75 mL intramuscularly once every two weeks. How many grams of the drug will the patient inject over the course of one year?

Practice Problem Answers
1. 128 fluid ounces
2. LX teaspoons
3. 8 tablespoons
4. 4 scruples
5. 183 centimeters
6. 3.18 kilograms
7. 10 tablespoons
8. 0.375 milliliters
9. 6 mL
10. 40 mg
11. 3.9 g

When insurance companies are billed for prescriptions, the pharmacy technician and pharmacist are responsible for calculating the days' supply being dispensed. If you bill an insurance company for a days' supply less than that actually dispensed (e.g. dispense a 30-day supply of medication and bill the insurance as though it were a 10-day supply) the insurance company can issue a "charge-back" during an audit (i.e. the pharmacy would have to pay the insurance company back; may also be referred to as "recoupment" by insurance companies). The most commonly prescribed medications are available from the manufacturer in the form of tablets or capsules ("solid oral dosage forms"). In these cases, determining the days' supply is a simple one-step calculation.

Example Problems
What is the days' supply for a prescription of 30 tablets of Drug X with the instructions to take one tablet by mouth once daily?

$$\frac{30 \text{ tablets}}{1} \times \frac{\text{day}}{1 \text{ tablet}} = 30 \text{ days}$$

What is the days' supply for a prescription of 60 tablets of Drug AB9012 with the instructions to take one tablet three times daily as needed for pain?

$$\frac{60 \text{ tablets}}{1} \times \frac{\text{day}}{3 \text{ tablets}} = 20 \text{ days}$$

Note: When the instructions include the term "as needed," assume the patient will use the maximum amount when calculating the days' supply.

Calculating the days' supply of a non-solid dosage form (e.g. oral liquids, eye drops, ear drops, nasal sprays, and inhalers) can be more challenging. Study the example problems on the next two pages, then practice these calculations yourself until you master them!

When necessary, use this information to complete the problems in this section:
ProAir®, Proventil®, and Ventolin® each contain 120 puffs/inhaler
Astepro® nasal spray contains 200 sprays/bottle
Flonase® nasal spray contains 120 sprays/bottle
Xalatan® eye drops contain 2.5 mL/bottle

More Example Problems

How many days will a 4-ounce bottle of cetirizine 5 mg/5 mL solution last if the instructions are to take one-half teaspoonful QHS?

Note: Make sure you read the question carefully!

$$\frac{120 \text{ mL}}{\text{bottle}} \times \frac{\text{tsp}}{5 \text{ mL}} \times \frac{\text{day}}{0.5 \text{ tsp}} = 48 \text{ days/bottle}$$

What would the days' supply be on a prescription for Flonase® nasal spray if the instructions are 1 spray in each nostril QD?

$$\frac{120 \text{ sprays}}{\text{bottle}} \times \frac{\text{day}}{2 \text{ sprays}} = 60 \text{ days/bottle}$$

Try it yourself: Calculate the days' supply of 1 bottle of Astepro® if the instructions say to instill 1 spray into each nostril BID.

Answer: 50 day-supply

A prescription is written for 3 Ventolin® HFA Inhalers with the instructions to inhale 2 puffs PO Q4-6H PRN wheezing. Each inhaler contains enough medication for 200 puffs. What would the days' supply of this prescription be?

$$\frac{3 \text{ inhalers}}{1} \times \frac{200 \text{ puffs}}{\text{inhaler}} \times \frac{\text{day}}{12 \text{ puffs}} = 50 \text{ days}$$

Test Your Knowledge

How many drops are in one milliliter (1 mL)?

Between 15 and 20 drops.

Note: In general, you should calculate days' supply based on 20 drops/mL, but the actual number of drops in one milliliter can vary based on the temperature, the density of the liquid in question, and other factors.

What is the days' supply for a 7.5 mL bottle of Ciprodex® Otic Solution with the instructions: ii gtts AS QID until gone?
   A.   7 days
   B.   10 days
   C.   12 days
   D.   19 days
   E.   25 days

Solution:

Step 1: *Interpret the sig.*

"ii gtts AS QID until gone"
   = instill two drops into the left ear four times daily until gone.

Step 2: *Since the question does not specify how many drops are in one milliliter, calculate the days' supply based on the conversion factor of 20 drops/mL.*

$$\frac{7.5\ \text{mL}}{1} \times \frac{20\ \text{drops}}{\text{mL}} \times \frac{\text{day}}{8\ \text{drops}} = 18.75\ \text{days} \therefore 19\ \text{days}$$

Answer: D. 19 days

You are dispensing a 5-mL bottle of ciprofloxacin 0.3% ophthalmic solution with instructions to instill two drops into each eye three times daily until gone. What is the days' supply of this prescription (assume 20 drops/mL)?

$$\frac{5\ \text{mL}}{1} \times \frac{20\ \text{drops}}{\text{mL}} \times \frac{\text{day}}{12\ \text{drops}} = 8\ \text{days}$$

The Rule of Hand
One (1) gram of topical medication is roughly enough to cover one side (palm and fingers) of four flat hands. Use the Rule of Hand when calculating the days' supply of topical medications.

Practice Problems

1. What is the days' supply for a 15-gram tube of acne medication with instructions to apply to the entire face nightly?
(Note: The area of the face is roughly equal to the area of two flat hands)

2. You are dispensing two Ventolin® HFA inhalers with instructions for the patient to inhale one to two puffs by mouth every four to six hours as needed for shortness of breath. What will the days' supply be for this prescription?

3. What is the days' supply for a quantity of 60 venlafaxine ER 37.5 mg capsules with the following instructions: i PO QD x 7 days, then i PO BID x 7 days, then ii QAM and i QPM thereafter?

4. What is the days' supply for a 120-mL bottle of Tussionex® suspension with the following instructions: take i tsp PO up to TID PRN for cough?

5. You dispense a prescription for methotrexate 2.5 mg tablets with instructions to take three tablets by mouth weekly. What is the days' supply for 30 tablets?

6. NovoLog® FlexPen is available in a package that contains five pens. Each pen contains three milliliters of NovoLog® insulin. If a patient uses 11 units SQ every morning and 9 units SQ every evening with a meal, what is the days' supply for a single package that contains five pens?
(Note: the concentration of NovoLog® insulin is 100 units per milliliter)

7. Antipyrine-benzocaine otic solution comes in a 15-mL bottle. What is the days' supply if the instructions are as follows: instill 2-4 gtts AU up to QID PRN?
(Note: Assume there are 20 drops per mL)

Practice Problem Answers
1. 30 days
2. 33 days
3. 27 days
4. 8 days
5. 70 days
6. 75 days
7. 9 days

Density (δ) = mass (grams) per unit volume (milliliters).

$$\text{Density} = \frac{\text{Mass (g)}}{\text{Volume(mL)}}$$

Specific gravity = the density of a substance relative to the density of a reference substance*.

$$\text{Specific Gravity} = \frac{\text{Density of Substance}}{\text{Density of Reference Substance}}$$

*The reference substance is almost always H_2O (water), which has a density of 1 g/mL. When this is the case, the specific gravity of a substance is the same value as the density but without the units. For example, the density of glycerin is 1.26 g/mL. When you calculate the specific gravity of glycerin, you take the density of glycerin and divide it by the density of water (1.26 g/mL ÷ 1 g/mL = 1.26). Essentially all that happens is the units cancel out, and you get specific gravity of glycerin = 1.26.

Example Problems
You weigh 30 mL of a mystery substance to determine its identity. If the 30 mL sample of the substance weighs 33.3 grams, what is the identity of the substance?

    A. Water (density = 1. 0 g/mL)
    B. Isopropyl Alcohol (density = 0.79 g/mL)
    C. Glycerin (density = 1.26 g/mL)
    D. Simple Syrup (density = 1.3 g/mL)
    E. Ethylene Glycol (density = 1.11 g/mL)

Solution:

$$\text{Density} = \frac{\text{Mass(g)}}{\text{Volume(mL)}}$$

$$\therefore \text{Density} = \frac{33.3\ g}{30\ mL} = 1.11\,g/mL$$

Answer: E. Ethylene Glycol (Density = 1.11 g/mL)

To compound 60 grams of a formulation that contains 10% (w/w) petrolatum, how many milliliters of pure melted liquid petrolatum would be required? (Note: Density of petrolatum = 0.9 g/mL)

Solution:

$$\frac{10 \text{ g petrolatum}}{100 \text{ g total}} \times \frac{60 \text{ g total formulation}}{1} = 6 \text{ g petrolatum}$$

$$\frac{6 \text{ g petrolatum}}{1} \times \frac{mL}{0.9 \text{ g}} = 6.67 \text{ mL petrolatum}$$

Answer: 6.67 mL of petrolatum

Practice Problems

1. How much does 4 mL of a substance weigh if its density is 1.2 g/mL?

2. What volume of simple syrup (density 1.3 g/mL) would be needed to obtain a sample that weighs 2 grams?

3. What would the specific gravity of water be (density = 1 g/mL) if the reference substance was glycerin (density = 1.26 g/mL)?

4. If 78 mL of Substance H weighs 131 grams, what is the density of Substance H?

5. If 12 grams of Liquid Q occupies a volume of 15 mL, what is the specific gravity of Liquid Q (assume reference substance is water)?

Practice Problem Answers
1. 4.8 g
2. 1.54 mL
3. 0.79
4. 1.68 g/mL
5. 0.8

A temperature conversion problem will be easy points on the PTCB exam provided that you know how to solve it. Memorize the equations for converting Fahrenheit to Celsius and Celsius to Fahrenheit and know how to apply them.

Converting from Fahrenheit to Celsius:

$$^{\circ}C = \frac{5}{9}(^{\circ}F - 32)$$

Converting from Celsius to Fahrenheit:

$$^{\circ}F = \left(\frac{9}{5} \times {}^{\circ}C\right) + 32$$

****

Temperature Conversion Values to Memorize
0°C = 32°F (freezing point of water)
37°C = 98.6°F (human body temperature)
100°C = 212°F (boiling point of water)

****

Example Problem
You read that insulin should be stored at 2 – 8°C. What is this temperature range in degrees Fahrenheit?

Solution:

$$\left(\frac{9}{5} \times 2^{\circ}C\right) + 32 = 36^{\circ}F \qquad \left(\frac{9}{5} \times 8^{\circ}C\right) + 32 = 46^{\circ}F$$

Answer: 36 – 46°F

Practice Problems
Convert the following temperature to degrees Fahrenheit:

1) -3°C
2) 0°C
3) 1°C
4) 6°C
5) 25°C
6) 60°C

Convert the following temperatures to degrees Celsius:

7) -10°F
8) 0°F
9) 32°F
10) 98.6°F
11) 72°F
12) 101°F

Practice Problem Answers
1) 27°F
2) 32°F
3) 34°F
4) 43°F
5) 77°F
6) 140°F
7) -23°C
8) -18°C
9) 0°C
10) 37°C
11) 22°C
12) 38.3°C

Weight-based dosing always requires the patient's weight to be in units of kilograms (kg). Here in the United States, we typically measure a person's weight in terms of pounds, not kilograms. For this reason, converting a patient's weight from pounds to kilograms will usually be the first step in calculating a weight-based dose. A lot of scenarios involve converting a patient's weight from pounds to kilograms, so it is extremely important that you master this calculation. Fortunately, the calculation is simple. Just remember that 1 kg = 2.2 lbs, and get a lot of practice by working through the examples and practice problems.

Infliximab is prescribed to a patient at the dose of 5 mg/kg. The patient weighs 154 pounds. How many milligrams of infliximab should be dispensed as one dose?

$$\frac{154 \text{ pounds}}{1} \times \frac{1 \text{ kg}}{2.2 \text{ pounds}} \times \frac{5 \text{ mg}}{\text{kg}} = 350 \text{ mg}$$

You calculate the appropriate dose of infliximab to be 350 mg. The dose is going to be administered IV in 250 mL of 0.9% NaCl. Infliximab comes in a vial containing 100 mg/20 mL solution. <u>How many vials</u> will you need to <u>open</u> in order to fill this prescription?

Answer: 4 vials (you will only use 3.5 vials-worth of the drug, but you will need to open 4 vials since you cannot open half of a vial)

How many milliliters of the drug solution will be needed to obtain 350 mg of infliximab for the aforementioned prescription?

$$\frac{350 \text{ mg}}{1} \times \frac{20 \text{ mL}}{100 \text{ mg}} = 70 \text{ mL}$$

Vancomycin is being dosed at 15 mg/kg for a patient that weighs 241 pounds and has a fever. How many milliliters of vancomycin 1 gram/20 mL solution will be needed to compound this prescription?

$$\frac{241 \text{ pounds}}{1} \times \frac{1 \text{ kg}}{2.2 \text{ pounds}} \times \frac{15 \text{ mg}}{\text{kg}} \times \frac{20 \text{ mL}}{1 \text{ g}} \times \frac{1 \text{ g}}{1,000 \text{ mg}} = 32.9 \text{ mL}$$

<u>Note</u>: Frequently you will receive problems that contain irrelevant information (in this case, the fact that the patient has a fever). Don't be distracted by this type of information; just move on and solve the problem using the relevant information.

Formula for Body Surface Area (BSA):

$$BSA = \sqrt{\frac{height\ (cm) \times weight\ (kg)}{3,600}}$$

What types of medications are typically dosed based on body surface area?
Cancer chemotherapy drugs.

What is the BSA of a patient that is 5 feet and 4 inches tall and weighs 110 pounds?

$$\sqrt{\frac{64\ inches}{1} \times \frac{2.54\ cm}{inch} \times \frac{110\ lbs}{1} \times \frac{1\ kg}{2.2\ lbs} \times \frac{1}{3,600}} = 1.50\ m^2$$

Note: BSA is expressed in units of square meters (m²).

The appropriate dose of Doxorubicin is 550 mg/m². How many milligrams are required to provide three doses to a male patient 6' 1" tall weighing 225 lbs?

$$\frac{73\ inches}{1} \times \frac{2.54\ cm}{inch} = 185\ cm \qquad \frac{225\ lbs}{1} \times \frac{1\ kg}{2.2\ lbs} = 102\ kg$$

$$\left(\sqrt{\frac{185\ cm \times 102\ kg}{3600}}\right) \times \frac{550\ mg}{m^2} \times \frac{3\ doses}{1} = 3777\ mg$$

Note: When you convert the height and weight to the metric system separately (as was done above) and then plug the numbers into the equation for BSA, your final answer will be slightly less accurate due to rounding. For this reason, it is better to calculate the height and weight and plug the values in all in one step (see below for example).

$$\left(\sqrt{\frac{73\ in}{1} \times \frac{2.54\ cm}{in} \times \frac{225\ lb}{1} \times \frac{1\ kg}{2.2\ lb} \times \frac{1}{3600}}\right) \times \frac{550\ mg}{m^2} \times \frac{3}{1} = 3787\ mg$$

This answer is more accurate, since the converted weight and height were not rounded.
In this case, there were only 2 significant figures, so technically the correct answer is 3,800 mg. Thus, both approaches yield the same answer for all practical purposes; however, it is always best to use the most accurate approach when solving math problems and then round your final answer up or down as necessary.

To determine the drip rate of an infusion, you must first identify the volume (i.e. the number of milliliters) that will be infused into the patient and the length of time over which the infusion will take place. Once you know the volume that needs to be infused per unit time, all you need to do is convert the volume from milliliters to drops based on how many drops per milliliter the administration set delivers (e.g. a microdrip administration set delivers 60 drops/mL). Then you will have your answer. It is simple unit conversion – take the given information and convert the units until you get the drip rate (drops/minute).

Test Your Knowledge
How many drops are there in one milliliter?
Typically there are 15-20 drops per milliliter, but droppers or infusion administration sets can be calibrated to deliver a just about any number of drops per milliliter (e.g. 10 drops/mL, 15 drops/mL, 20 drops/mL, 60 drops/mL).

Some IV administration sets deliver 60 drops/mL, what are these called?
Microdrip administration sets.

Example Problems
A 500 mL solution contains 2 grams of Drug X. How many mL/minute should be administered for the patient to receive 200 mg/hour?

Solution:
Step 1: *Determine the concentration of the infusion solution.*
$$\frac{2\,\text{grams}}{500\,\text{mL}} \times \frac{1{,}000\,\text{mg}}{\text{gram}} = 4\,\text{mg/mL}$$

Step 2: *Calculate the infusion rate in units of mL/min.*
$$\frac{200\,\text{mg}}{\text{hr}} \times \frac{\text{mL}}{4\,\text{mg}} \times \frac{\text{hr}}{60\,\text{min}} = 0.83\,\text{mL/min}$$

Answer: 0.83 mL/min

In the problem above, what would the drip rate be if a drip set that delivers 60 drops/mL is utilized?

Solution:

$$\frac{0.83\,\text{mL}}{\text{min}} \times \frac{60\,\text{drops}}{\text{mL}} = 50\,\text{drops/min}$$

Answer: 50 drops/min

A patient is receiving 15,000 units of heparin per hour from an IV bag containing 250 mL of 100 unit/mL heparin. If the administration set delivers 20 drops/mL, how many drops is the patient receiving each minute?

Solution:

$$\frac{15{,}000 \text{ units}}{\text{hr}} \times \frac{\text{mL}}{100 \text{ units}} \times \frac{20 \text{ drops}}{\text{mL}} \times \frac{\text{hr}}{60 \text{ min}} = 50 \text{ drops/min}$$

Answer: 50 drops/min

Milrinone is being dosed at 0.33 mcg/kg/min for a 210 lb patient with a creatinine clearance of 30 mL/min. The infusion bag contains Milrinone 40 mg in 200 mL of D5W. What is the drip rate if a microdrip administration set (60 drops/min) is being used?

Solution:

$$\frac{0.33 \text{ mcg}}{\text{kg} \bullet \text{min}} \times \frac{210 \text{ lb}}{1} \times \frac{\text{kg}}{2.2 \text{ lb}} \times \frac{200 \text{ mL}}{40 \text{ mg}} \times \frac{1 \text{ mg}}{1{,}000 \text{ mcg}} \times \frac{60 \text{ drops}}{\text{mL}} = 9 \text{ drops/min}$$

Answer: 9 drops/min

A physician orders Vasopressin 30 milliunits/min. You dispense a 250-mL sterile admixture containing 25 units of Vasopressin in normal saline. If the administration set delivers 20 drops per minute, what is the appropriate drip rate?

Solution:

$$\frac{30 \text{ milliunits}}{\text{min}} \times \frac{250 \text{ mL}}{25 \text{ units}} \times \frac{\text{unit}}{1{,}000 \text{ milliunits}} \times \frac{20 \text{ drops}}{\text{mL}} = 6 \text{ drops/min}$$

Answer: 6 drops/min

Practice Problems

1. What is the drip rate for a 250-mL bag of Vancomycin 1g in NSS if it is infused over one hour using a microdrip administration set (60 drops/milliliter)?

2. An administration set delivering 30 drops/mL was used to infuse a 160-mL bag of magnesium sulfate solution over the course of 120 minutes. What was the drip rate in units of drops/minute?

3. Drug M is available as a 100 mcg/1 mL infusion. If the patient receiving this infusion weighs 176 pounds and Drug M is being dosed at 10 mcg/kg/hr, what should the drip rate be if a microdrip administration set is used?

4. A patient receives 1 liter of Drug P over 24 hours. What is the drip rate if an administration set that delivers 19 drops/mL is used?

Practice Problem Answers
1. 250 drops/minute
2. 40 drops/minute
3. 8 drops/minute
4. 13 drops/minute

What are the three major methods for calculating pediatric doses based on adult dosing information?

1. Clark's Rule
2. Young's Rule
3. BSA dosing

Clark's Rule

$$\text{Child Dose} = \frac{\text{Child's Weight (lbs)}}{150 \text{ lbs}} \times \text{Adult Dose}$$

What is the significance of the value 150 lbs?
150 lbs is the average adult weight.

Young's Rule

$$\text{Child Dose} = \frac{\text{Child's Age}}{(\text{Child's Age} + 12)} \times \text{Adult Dose}$$

BSA Dosing

$$\text{Child Dose} = \frac{\text{Child's BSA}}{1.73 \text{ m}^2} \times \text{Adult Dose}$$

What is the significance of the value 1.73 m²?
1.73 m² is the average adult body surface area (BSA).

Example Problems
You are dispensing a prescription for prednisone for a 6-year-old patient that is 3′ 5″ tall and weighs 49 pounds. What is the appropriate pediatric dose for this patient based on BSA dosing if the adult dose is 20 mg?

Solution:

$$\text{Child Dose} = \dfrac{\sqrt{\dfrac{41\text{ in}}{1} \times \dfrac{2.54\text{ cm}}{\text{in}} \times \dfrac{49\text{ lbs}}{1} \times \dfrac{\text{kg}}{2.2\text{ lbs}}}{3,600}}{1.73\text{ m}^2} \times 20\text{ mg} = 9.3\text{ mg}$$

Answer: 9.3 mg

What is the appropriate dose based on Young's Rule?

Solution:

$$\text{Child Dose} = \dfrac{6}{(6+12)} \times 20\text{ mg} = 6.7\text{ mg}$$

Answer: 6.7 mg

What is the appropriate dose based on Clark's Rule?

Solution:

$$\text{Child Dose} = \dfrac{49\text{ lbs}}{150\text{ lbs}} \times 20\text{ mg} = 6.5\text{ mg}$$

Answer: 6.5 mg

Using Clark's Rule, calculate the appropriate dose of Drug X for a 30 kg child (the adult dose is 750 mg).

A. 150 mg
B. 250 mg
C. 300 mg
D. 330 mg
E. 460 mg

Solution:

$$\text{Child Dose} = \frac{\left(\dfrac{30 \text{ kg}}{1} \times \dfrac{2.2 \text{ lbs}}{\text{kg}}\right)}{150 \text{ lbs}} \times 750 \text{ mg} = 330 \text{ mg}$$

Answer: D. 330 mg

Note: Never overlook what units you are working with. If you forget to convert the patient's weight from kilograms to pounds before using Clark's Rule, you will miss questions like this.

Practice Problems

1. The adult dose of Drug HD3021 is 400 mg once daily. What is the appropriate dose of Drug HD3021 for a 10-year-old male child that is 53 inches tall and weighs 78 pounds? Use Clark's Rule.

2. The adult dose of a drug is 150 mg twice daily for three days. How many milligrams (for a three-day course of therapy) should be dispensed to an 8-year-old female child that is 45 inches tall and weighs 57 pounds? Use Young's Rule.

3. Based on an adult dose of 600 mg, what is the appropriate dose for a 6-year-old boy that is 3 feet 4 inches tall and weighs 44 pounds? Use BSA Dosing.

4. If the adult dose if a drug is 1 gram, what is the appropriate dose for an 11-year-old child that weighs 100 pounds? Use Clark's Rule.

5. If the adult dose if a drug is 1 gram, what is the appropriate dose for an 11-year-old child that weighs 100 pounds? Use Young's Rule.

Practice Problem Answers

1. 208 mg
2. 360 mg (60 mg per dose x 6 doses)
3. 260 mg
4. 667 mg
5. 478 mg

The human body naturally produces steroid hormones. Taking steroids medicinally leads to a reduction in the body's internal production of steroids. At high doses, use of medicinal steroids can shut down steroid hormone production within the body entirely. For this reason, when discontinuing high doses of steroids, it is necessary to decrease the dose gradually over time (as opposed to abruptly stopping the medication) to give the body time to turn steroid production back on. This process of gradual reduction is called a taper.

When doctors prescribe short courses of a high-dose steroid, they will often use a dose pack. An example of a steroid dose pack is the prednisone 10 mg 6-day dose pack where the patient takes 6 tablets the first day and decreases by one tablet daily until finished (6, 5, 4, 3, 2, 1, stop). With dose packs, the manufacturer includes the instructions directly on the packaging. This makes it more convenient for the patient and the prescriber.

It should be noted that steroid tapers can be accomplished without the use of a dose pack. For instance, a prescriber could issue a prescription for prednisone with instructions to take 30 mg daily for 3 days, 20 mg daily for 3 days, 10 mg daily for 3 days, 5 mg daily for 3 days, and then stop.

Note: The term "taper" can also be used to describe gradually increasing the dose of a medication (also known as "titrating" the dose). Starting at a low dose and increasing it slowly up to the optimal therapeutic dose allows the body to gradually build a tolerance to the drug, thus reducing the incidence of side effects. For example, gabapentin is often initiated at a low dose and then gradually increased to a more effective dose in an attempt to avoid the side effect of drowsiness. Another example is metformin, which is usually dosed in a similar fahion to avoid side effects such as upset stomach and diarrhea.

When dealing with tapers, days' supply calculations can be more challenging. Remember, when an insurance company is improperly billed for a prescription, they can recoup previously paid money in an audit; in other words, the pharmacy must pay them back. For instance, if an insurance company audits your pharmacy and finds that a prescription was dispensed for a 90-day supply, but you billed them as though the prescription were only a 30-day supply, the insurance company can say that the claim was not submitted correctly and demand that the pharmacy pay them back.

Useful Fact: 5 mg and 10 mg prednisone dose packs are available in a 48 tablet 6-day dose pack and a 21 tablet 12-day dose pack.

While we are on the topic, let's talk about the term "dosepak." Some people use the terms "dosepak" and "dose pack" interchangeably. Truth be told, "dosepak" is not a real word; rather, it is a portion of one of Pfizer's brand name drugs, the Medrol® Dosepak™. The name is similar to one of Pfizer's other inventions, the Z-pak®. The names ending in "pak" belong to Pfizer. All other dose packs (such as prednisone dose packs, generic methylprednisolone dose packs, and generic azithromycin dose packs) are just called "dose packs."

KNOWLEDGE DOMAIN #7
PHARMACY INVENTORY MANAGEMENT
(8.75% OF EXAM)

NDC stands for "National Drug Code." An NDC number is an 11-digit number that is divided into 3 parts. The first part identifies <u>who</u> manufactured the product, the second part identifies <u>what</u> the product is, and the third part is typically used to identify the <u>size</u> of the package or the quantity of dosage units contained in the package. The format of an NDC number is as follows:

Structure of an NDC Number

12345-1234-12

First Segment (5 digits)
The first 5 number segment of the NDC number identifies the manufacturer of a product (e.g. 00093 is the 5-digit code for TEVA, 52544 represents Watson).

Second Segment (4 digits)
The middle 4 number segment of the NDC number identifies the product made by the manufacturer (e.g. 0913 is Watson Pharmaceutical's 4-digit code for Norco® 5/325 mg).

Third Segment (2 digits)
The ending 2 number segment of the NDC number usually identifies the package size of the product (e.g. the NDC number for a 100 tablet bottle of Watson's Norco® 5/325 mg is 52544-0913-<u>01</u> and the NDC number for a 500 tablet bottle is 52544-0913-<u>05</u>).

<u>Note</u>: Frequently, a trailing zero is omitted from the NDC number displayed on the label of the manufacturer's stock bottle. For instance, the 11-digit NDC 00093-0287-01 would typically be displayed on the stock bottle in one of the following three formats:

0093-0287-01

00093-287-01

00093-0287-1

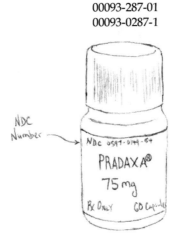

Are *all* drug products required to have a lot number?
All drug products must have a lot number assigned by the manufacturer. A different lot number is assigned to each batch of a drug product produced. So, all drugs from the same production batch share the same lot number.

What is the purpose of the lot number?
Lot numbers play an important role in drug manufacturing and pharmacy practice. If a drug product has an abnormality, such as discoloration or contamination, the lot number is used to identify and recall the affected batch.

What happens if a drug product has no lot number (e.g. the label was torn and the lot number is no longer visible or identifiable)?
During a recall, containers of a drug product that are missing a lot number must be treated as though they are in the recalled batch.

Do all prescription drugs have an expiration date?
Yes, the FDA requires manufacturers to assign expiration dates for all prescription drugs.

Is it alright to use a drug product that is expired?
The expiration date is the final date through which the manufacturer can guarantee the potency and safety of the drug. Use of an expired drug cannot be recommended.

Let's say that the label on a drug label indicates an expiration date of 08/2018. Will the drug be expired on 08/02/2018?
No, the drug will be expired on the final day of 08/2018, which would be 08/31/2018.

The date is July 19, 2015. The expiration date on a vial of insulin is 09/31/2016. The stopper of this vial of insulin was initially punctured on June 18, 2015. The insulin will be expired after which day?
    A. 06/18/2015
    B. 07/16/2015
    C. 07/18/2015
    D. 09/31/2016

    Answer:
    B. 07/16/2015
    Since the expiration date printed on the vial is 09/31/2016, the rubber stopper of the vial may be first punctured for use up to 09/31/2016; however, once punctured the contents of the vial only remain sterile for 28 days. Twenty-eight days from 06/18/2015 would be 07/16/2015.

Maintain Par Levels

The par level is the minimum quantity of a drug (or other product) that must be kept on-hand to meet the day-to-day needs of a business. For instance, if you normally dispense 600 tablets of lisinopril 20 mg per day, then the par level for that drug should be set to around 600 tablets. To ensure the inventory is sufficient to support normal day-to-day business operations, you need to keep track of how much inventory you have on-hand. When the inventory of a particular drug or product falls below the par level, an order to replenish the inventory must be placed. Most pharmacies utilize an automated inventory replenishment system. In these cases, the par level is programmed in the computer, and when the computerized inventory record indicates that the inventory for a particular drug or product falls below the par level, an order is automatically placed through the computer.

Rotate Stock

When a pharmacy receives a shipment of medications from a distributor or manufacturer, the pharmacy technician places each medication in its assigned location on the shelf (usually in alphabetical order). When placing newly received items on the shelf, it is important to "rotate stock." In other words, place the newer items toward the back of the shelf and move the older items to the front. This is done to ensure that the older medications are used first, thus reducing the chance of accumulating expired medications. Expired medications are ineffective, potentially unsafe, and should promptly be removed from the shelves.

Hospital Formulary

Instead of managing an overly large, overly diverse inventory of medications, hospitals use a preferred drug list, or "formulary," to determine which medications will be maintained on-hand. For instance, there are several ACE inhibitors on the market, but they all do pretty much the same thing. Rather than try to maintain an inventory that includes every ACE inhibitor, a hospital pharmacy may decide to only keep lisinopril and ramipril in stock. When a patient that has been taking a different ACE inhibitor (e.g. quinapril) is admitted to the hospital, the doctor switches the patient's medication to one of the options from the formulary (lisinopril or ramipril). Who determines which drugs to place on the hospital formulary? These decisions are made by a formulary team composed of physicians, pharmacists, nurses, and other healthcare professionals.

Most prescription medications have specific storage requirements or manufacturer-recommended storage conditions that must be met to ensure the product remains stable and effective until the assigned expiration date. Many environmental factors can negatively affect the chemical structure of the active ingredient(s) and/or disrupt the physical properties of the medium used to deliver the drug into the body (e.g. the drug delivery device and/or the inactive ingredients used to formulate the drug product). The most common examples of these deleterious environmental factors are:

- Temperature
    - Temperature can destroy the chemical and physical properties of a drug product. Study the chart below to learn how terms used in a manufacturer's product packaging like "keep cool" or "store at room temperature" can be translated into quantitative temperature ranges.
- Humidity/Moisture
    - Humidity and moisture can also destroy the chemical and physical properties of a drug product. Study the chart below to learn how terms used in product packaging like "store in a dry place" or "protect from moisture" can be translated into quantitative values.
- Sunlight
    - Sunlight is rich in ultraviolet (UV) light, which has the capcity to change the chemical structure of the active and inactive ingredients that make up the drug product. This is why pharmacies use amber vials/containers to dispense medications.

Temperature Ranges	
"Frozen" (Freezer)	-25°C to -10°C (-13°F to 14°F)
"Cold" (Refrigerator)	2°C to 8°C (36°F to 46°F)
"Cool"	8°C to 15°C (46°F to 59°F)
"Room Temperature"	20°C to 25°C (68°F to 77°F)
"Warm"	30°C to 40°C (86°F to 104°F)
"Excessive Heat"	> 40°C (> 104°F)

Humidity Ranges	
"Store in a Dry Place"	Average Relative Humidity < or = 40%
"Protect from Moisture"	Relative Humidity < or = 60%*

*Defined by the World Health Organization (WHO) Technical Report Series.

Drugs with Special Storage Requirements – Select Examples:

Product	Special Storage Requirement
Nitrostat® (nitroglycerin sublingual tablets)	Do not remove tablets from original container. Nitrogylcerin is a volatile substance that can quickly convert to a gaseous state. When stored outside of the original container, the nitroglycerin will evaporate from the tablet. For this reason, it is important to store nitroglycerin tablets tightly sealed in the original container (usually a small glass vial with a metal screw-on lid).
Pradaxa® (dabigatran oral capsules)	Pradaxa® is available in a bottle or blister packs. For the bottle, it is important to not remove any capsule from from original container until immediately prior to use. The drug is quickly destroyed by humidity in the air. The Pradaxa® bottle is equipped with a special cap that contains a dessicant (drying agent). Once the bottle is opened, the capsules inside will expire after 4 months. For the blister packs, do not remove a capsule from the blister pack until immediately prior to use.
Xalatan® (latanoprost eye drops)	Refrigerate (2° – 8^oC) until opened. Once opened, latanoprost eye drops can be stored at room temperature (up to 25^oC) for 6 weeks.
Insulin (all types and brands)	Refrigerate (2° – 8^oC) until first use; once the rubber stopper of the insulin vial is punctured, it can be stored either in the refrigerator or at room temperature for up to 28 days. After 28 days, sterility cannot be guaranteed.
Nitropress® (sodium nitroprusside injection)	Sodium nitroprusside is quickly deactivated upon exposure to light. To prevent the drug from being exposed to light, the medication comes in a small box. Each box contains a dark amber glass vial of sodium nitroprusside 50 mg/2 mL solution and an opaque light protective sleeve. The vial should only be removed from the box just prior to admixture. Once admixed, the IV infusion bag containing sodium nitroprusside must be placed in the opaque light protective sleeve to prevent exposure to light.

Consequences of Inappropriate Storage – Select Examples:

Product	Consequence
Aerosols *Inhalers* - ProAir®, Ventolin®, Xopenex®, Qvar®, Symbicort®, Serevent®, Atrovent® *Rectal Aerosols* - ProctoFoam®, ProctoFoam®-HC *Topical Aerosols* - Kenalog® spray, Tinactin® powder spray	Excessive heat can cause an aerosol container to burst/explode. When used at cool or colder temperatures, aerosols canisters tend to deliver less medication (suboptimal drug delivery).
Insulin Levemir®, Lantus®, Humulin N®, Novolin N®, Humulin R®, Novolin R®, Humalog®, NovoLog®, Apidra® (and all other forms of insulin)	Insulin is a protein, which is a large molecule whose effectiveness is dependent upon its complex chemical structure. Proteins, such as insulin, have a rather delicate chemical structure. Temperature extremes (heat and cold) and physical shaking can destroy the chemical structure of proteins, rendering them inactive. Additionally, insulin is delivered as an injection in a sterile liquid medium. Warmth and excessive heat can promote microbial contamination of the liquid medium, rendering the preparation unsafe for injection.
Suppositories Anucort-HC™ suppositories, Canasa® suppositories, Phenadoz™ suppositories, Glycerin suppositories	A suppository should be maintained in its individual wrapping until directly prior to insertion to protect the dosage form from humidity and moisture in the surrounding environment. If unwrapped and stored, the suppositories can adhere to one another. Heat and moisture can cause the suppository to melt and lose form.
Ointments Bactroban® Ointment, Mycolog®-II Ointment, Cortizone-10® Ointment	Warm environments and excessive heat can cause product separation.

Note: The bathroom is one of the worst places to store medication. Why? Hot baths and/or showers create steam (remember that moisture and heat can destroy the active ingredient(s)).

KNOWLEDGE DOMAIN #8
PHARMACY BILLING AND REIMBURSEMENT
(8.75% OF EXAM)

What is "self-pay?"

"Self-pay" means the patient or customer pays the full cost of the prescription without the help of any third party payers. Depending on which forms of payment your pharmacy accepts, self-pay customers can pay for their prescription(s) using cash, credit card, personal check, etc.

What is a third party payer?

The term "third party payer" refers to an entity outside of the patient-pharmacist relationship that is involved in the financial transaction. The pharmacy is the first party in the transaction, the patient or customer is the second party, and in cases where insurance (or a manufacturer coupon or discount card) is involved, the insurance company is the referred to as the "third party."

What is an insurance claim?

An insurance claim is a request for the payment of a product or service. If the product or service is covered under the terms of the insurance policy, the insurance company will send the payment to the provider on behalf of the customer/patient.

What is an insurance premium?

An insurance premium is the cost of maintaining active insurance coverage; it is usually charged on a monthly basis or deducted from your paycheck if obtained through your employer. For instance, a company may charge $90/month to provide coverage.

What is a deductible?

A deductible is the amount of money a patient must pay out-of-pocket (in addition to the premium) before the insurance benefits take effect. For instance, let's say Plan A offers 80% co-insurance after a $3,000 annual deductible for a premium of $200/month. In this case, the patient has to record $3,000 worth of out-of-pocket medical expenses (not including the $200/month premium) before the 80% co-insurance takes effect. In other words, the patient pays 100% of the cost of medical expenses until costs reach $3,000. After costs reach $3,000, then isurance pays 80% of medical expenses. This cycle starts over at the beginning of each year.

Note: Typically insurance policies with a higher deductible have a lower premium and vice versa. For example, an insurance company might offer one policy with a $3,000 annual deductible at a premium of $200/month and another policy with a $1,500 annual deductible at a premium of $300/month. People that do not believe they will use their insurance can increase the deductible to lower their premium.

What is an insurance formulary?

An insurance formulary is a list of drugs covered by an insurance policy. With many formularies, covered drugs are categorized into tiers. For instance, cheaper and more effective drugs are listed in tier one and are associated with lower co-pays than the more expensive and less effective drugs listed in tiers two and three.

What is a co-payment?

A co-payment (or "co-pay") is an amount of money paid by the insured person in according to the terms of the insurance policy. For instance, a prescription drug insurance policy might require the patient to pay a $45 co-pay for brand name prescription drugs and a $10 co-pay for generic prescription drugs. For some plans, instead of charging a fixed dollar amount, the co-payment might be a percentage of the total cost (e.g. a 20% co-payment). As with a deductible, a co-payment is an expense that must be assumed by the patient in addition to the insurance premium.

What is an HMO?

An HMO (Health Maintenance Organization) is a type of managed care insurance plan. Managed care plans work by forming agreements with healthcare providers. In the agreement, providers agree to certain treatment guidelines and reimbursement rates set by the HMO. When a provider's services are covered by an HMO insurance plan, the patients with those plans are more likely to use that provider's services. So, the prescriber benefits by getting to see more patients.

What is a PPO?

A PPO (Preferred Provider Organization) is another type of managed care insurance plan. Like an HMO, a PPO covers medical expenses incurred from healthcare providers and hospitals that have entered into a contract with the PPO. As with an HMO, the provider agrees to certain treatment guidelines and reimbursement rates. Patients that have that PPO coverage are more likely to visit a covered provider, so the provider benefits from the agreement by getting to see more patients.

What is CMS?

CMS (Centers for Medicare & Medicaid Services) is the division of the United States Department of Health & Human Services (DHHS) that is responsible for the administration of government health insurance programs such as Medicare, Medicaid, and SCHIP (State Children's Health Insurance Program).

What is Medicare?

Medicare is a federally funded health insurance program that covers the elderly (age 65 years and older), people under age 65 with certain disabilities, and people of any age with certain types of kidney disease. There are 4 parts of Medicare: Part A, Part B, Part C, and Part D. Part A is hospitalization insurance. Part B covers outpatient medical services, durable medical equipment (e.g. wheelchairs), preventive services (e.g. vaccines), supplies needed to diagnoses and treat medical conditions (e.g. blood glucose test strips and lancets for patients with diabetes), and certain medications that are not typically self-administered (e.g. oral cancer chemotherapy drugs and immunosuppressants). Part C plans are *optional* and are referred to as "medicare advantage plans." Part C provides the option to have your Part A & Part B coverage administered by a private insurance company rather than the federal government. Part D is *optional* prescription drug coverage. Part D is administered by private insurance companies, unlike Part A & Part B, which are administered directly by the federal government.

What is Medicaid?
Medicaid is health insurance/prescription drug insurance for people of any age with low-income and insufficient resources. Funding for Medicaid is provided by federal and state governments.

Note: Some people qualify for both Medicare *and* Medicaid.

What is a prior authorization?
When an insurance company requires a "prior authorization," they will not agree to pay the claim until they hear why the prescriber has chosen the drug that was prescribed. Usually prior authorizations are required when the prescribed drug is expensive and cheaper alternatives with similar effectiveness exist. When an insurance company requires prior authorization, the pharmacy's role is simply to notify the prescriber that a prior authorization is required. Then the prescriber must contact the inurance company. It is the prescriber's responsibility to complete a prior authorization – it is not up to the pharmacy. Typically, after the prescriber does their part, it takes the insurance company an additional 2 – 3 days to process the prior authorization. So, it is wise to inform the patient that the entire process may take several days.

What are some reasons an insurance claim might be rejected?
Rejections may occur for a variety of reasons. An insurance company may reject a claim for a number of reasons. Some examples are outlined below:

- NDC not covered
  - This type of rejection occurs when you try to bill an insurance plan for medications that are not on the formulary. Over-the-counter (OTC) drugs are often rejected for this reason.
- Refill too soon
- Therapeutic duplication
- Drug-drug interaction
- Drug utilization review (DUR)
  - Can be overridden if the pharmacist verifies the appropriateness of the prescription.
- Look-alike/sound-alike
  - Some insurance companies will initially reject claims for medications that have error-prone names (like hydralazine and hydroxyzine). This forces the pharmacist to take a closer look at the medication name, reducing the chance of a dispensing error.
- Dose too high
  - When you bill for a days' supply that is too short based on the amount of medication being dispensed and common prescribing practices, the insurance company may reject the claim until you verify the dose with the prescriber and document the discussion.

Note: When you contact a prescriber's office to clarify any part of a prescription, always document the following information on the prescription hardcopy:
1. The details that were verified or changed.
2. The name of the person you spoke to.
3. The date and time of the conversation.
4. Your name or initials.

What is a plan limitation?
Some insurance plans limit the quantity of a medication they will cover. For instance, a plan may only cover a maximum of 15 tablets of zolpidem in a 30-day time period. In these cases, if you try to bill the plan for 16 tablets or more for a 30-days' supply, the claim will be rejected.

What is a Pharmacy Benefits Manager (PBM)?
A Pharmacy Benefits Manager (PBM) is the administrator of the prescription drug portion of a health insurance plan. PBMs enter into contracts* with pharmacies, develop formularies, and process prescription drug claims.

*A pharmacy must be contracted with a patient's insurance company in order for the patient to use their insurance benefits at that particular pharmacy.

What is a Medication Assistance Program (MAP)?
A Medication Assistance Program (MAP) is a program that provides financial help for patients that cannot afford their medications.

How do prescription drug coupons work?
Prescription drug coupons must be billed just like insurance plans. Many patients present their drug coupons after the prescription has been filled. This can disrupt workflow since you have to process the third party claim again. To avoid disrupting workflow, ask the patient for any coupons at the time the prescription is first dropped off.

Note: Prescription drug coupons cannot be used by patients enrolled in government prescription drug insurance programs, such as Medicaid or Medicare Part D. Also, each coupon has its own fine print (terms & conditions) that may limit a patient's ability to use the coupon; for example, the fine print might indicate that the patient must be at least 18 years of age in order to use the coupon).

What is "coordination of benefits?"
The word "benefits" refers to multiple third party payers, so this applies to situations where a patient is covered by more than one third party payer. In these cases, each payer cannot be charged for the total claim. Each payer must be charged only for the amount that they are individually responsible for paying. Intentionally or unintentionally obtaining duplicate payments or payments in excess of 100% of the claim is an act of *insurance fraud*. Coordinating benefits means billing the third party payers in the correct order (e.g. charging the primary insurance first for the full price of the prescription and charging the the secondary insurance second for the co-payment).

What is home health care?
Home health care is just what it sounds like – delivery of health care directly in the patient's home. Usually this involves a nurse visiting the patient's home periodically for monitoring and administering medications. An example might be a patient with a bacterial infection of the bone (osteomyelitis) requiring several weeks of IV antibiotic therapy. The patient is initially diagnosed and treated in the hospital, but once stabilized, the patient is sent home to receive home health care (periodic monitoring and infusion of IV antibiotics) for the remaining few weeks of therapy. By receiving therapy at home rather than in the hospital, thousands of dollars in medical expenses are avoided and the patient's outcome is virtually the same.

What is a home infusion pharmacy?
A home infusion pharmacy is a pharmacy that prepares and delivers medications for administration in the patient's home. These pharmacies typically prepare things like PCA (patient controlled analgesia) pumps, IV antibiotics, IV electrolytes, IM vitamin B12, heparin flushes, TPNs*, and any other sterile parenteral formulations that might be administered in a patient's home.

*TPN stands for Total Parenteral Nutrition, which is a sterile mixture of nutrients (e.g. carbohydrates, proteins, fats, and vitamins) delivered by infusion into the bloodstream. Use of TPNs is reserved for critical cases in which a patient cannot cosume food/nutrients by normal means. What does "parenteral" mean? "Par-" comes from the Greek prefix "para-" meaning aside or beyond, and "-enteral," come from the Greek word for intestinal tract. So, if something is administered parenterally, that means it is delivered by a route other than the intestinal tract. Typically, "parenteral" is used to refer to formulations that are administered by intravenous infusion, though technically the word could also describe any method of delivery that avoids the gastrointestinal tract.

Dispense as written (DAW) codes are submitted as part of a third party claim (i.e. the DAW code is transmitted to the insurance company when the pharmacy bills for a prescription). The purpose of the DAW code is to describe why the generic form of the drug or the brand form was dispensed.

DAW 0 = generic substitution permitted by prescriber
DAW 1 = generic substitution not allowed by prescriber
DAW 2 = generic substitution permitted, but patient requested brand product
DAW 3 = generic substitution permitted, but pharmacist selected brand
DAW 4 = generic substitution permitted, but generic not in-stock
DAW 5 = generic substitution permitted, but brand dispensed as generic
DAW 6 = all-purpose override
DAW 7 = law mandated that the brand product be dispensed
DAW 8 = generic substitution permitted, but generic not available on the market
DAW 9 = other

Use the prescription below to answer the questions on the next page.

James Smith, D.O.
Simplified Medical Clinic • 10001 N. Main St. Suite 100A
Simple City, USA 24680
Telephone: (123) 555-1234

Name _John Doe_   Age **25**
Address _111 N. Main St. Anywhere, USA 10001_   Date **2-27-15**

Rx   Bactrim DS
    Disp. #20 tablets
    ⊤ PO BID x 10 days
    (NR)

NR	1	2	3	4	5	PRN

J. Smith , D.O.

Prescriber Must Write "Brand Name Medically Necessary" on the Prescription to Prohibit Generic Substitution.

You are billing John Doe's insurance for the Bactrim® DS prescription shown on the previous page. Since the doctor signed over the line that says "product selection permitted," you are going to dispense the generic (sulfamethoxazole 800 mg/ trimethoprim 160 mg). What DAW code should you enter for this prescription?
DAW 0.

John Doe leaves the pharmacy to go grocery shopping while his prescription is being filled. When he returns to the pharmacy to pick up his prescription, he insists on getting the brand name version of the medication. What DAW code would you submit to the insurance in this scenario?
DAW 2.

After Mr. Doe discovers that his insurance will not cover the brand name version of the medication, he tells you that he will go ahead and get the generic version. What DAW code would you submit to the insurance now?
DAW 0.

What DAW code would you enter for the prescription if the doctor had signed the line on the right instead of the line on the left?
When the doctor signs the "Dispense as Written" line, you must dispense the medication exactly as written (no generic substitution allowed). In this scenario, the correct answer is DAW 1.

What condition is Bactrim DS used to treat?
Bacterial infection.

What does the "DS" in Bactrim® DS stand for?
"DS" is an abbreviation for "double strength." Bactrim® is a combination drug, meaning that a single tablet contains two medications. In this case, the two medications are the antibioitics sulfamethoxazole and trimethoprim (sometimes abbreviated as SMZ/TMP). One dose of regular strength Bactrim® contains 400 mg of sulfamethoxazole and 80 mg of trimethoprim. Each dose of Bactrim® DS contains twice the amount of each active ingredient (800 mg of sulfamethoxazole and 160 mg of trimethoprim). Bactrim® and Bactrim® DS are also available under the brand name Septra® and Septra® DS.

What is Wholesale Acquisition Cost (WAC)?
WAC is the price a wholesaler would pay a manufacturer to purchase a drug.

Why is WAC important?
WAC is commonly used when pricing drugs items.

How is WAC used to price a drug item?
The amount the pharmacy charges the patient (retail cost) is typically determined using the following equation:

$$Retail\ Cost = WAC + Markup + Dispensing\ Fee$$

What is a dispensing fee?
A fee charged by the pharmacist to cover costs associated with filling the prescription (e.g. paying employee wages, recordkeeping, checking for drug interactions, providing advice and answering questions). A typical dispensing fee is about $2 - $12 per prescription.

Example Problems
What is the retail cost (cost to the customer) of Drug X if WAC is $49.56, the Markup is 20%, and the Dispensing Fee is $10?
Retail Cost = WAC + Markup + Dispensing Fee
Retail Cost = $49.55 + ($49.56 x 0.2) + $10 = $69.46

What would be the WAC for Drug Y if the Retail Cost is $9.00, the Dispensing Fee is $2.00, and the Markup is 25%?
WAC = Retail Cost – Dispensing Fee – Markup
WAC = $9.00 – $2.00 – ($7.00 x 0.25) = $5.60

Practice Problems
1. What is the Retail Cost of Drug B if WAC = $20, the dispensing fee = $8, and the markup is 50%?

2. What is the WAC of Drug C if the Retail Cost is $99.96, the Markup is 15%, and the Dispensing Fee is $7.50?

Practice Problem Answers
1. $38
2. $80.40

What is a pharmacy information system?
Pharmacy information systems are software programs used by pharmacy departments in institutional facilities (e.g. hospitals, long-term care facilities). Most pharmacy information systems function to help pharmacists accomplish the following:
- Receive and dispense orders via computerized physician order entry (CPOE).
- Receive and dispense e-prescriptions.
- Verify medication orders.
- Facilitate bar-coded drug administration.
- Maintain patient drug profiles (e.g. medication administration records, medication histories, allergy records).
- Access patient charts and lab results.
- Identify potential drug-related problems (e.g. drug interactions).
- Perform drug dose checking.
- Manage drug inventory.
- Purchase drugs from a distributor.
- Set prices and charge/bill for drugs.
- Generate reports (e.g. drug use evaluation reports, override reports).
- Maintain the confidentiality of patients' protected health information.

Note: When you have access to a pharmacy information system, *never* share your login information (i.e. password) with anyone, including your manager. When you are logged in, a digital fingerprint is left in every file visited under your name. If someone other than you creates a problem, such as a privacy violation, under your name on the computer you could face serious consequences.

What are the names of some commonly used pharmacy information systems?
- Meditech
- Horizon Meds Manager
- PharmNet
- Epic
- Siemens Pharmacy
- RxConnect
- Sunrise Pharmacy

How does a pharmacy information system keep track of inventory?
Whenever a medication is received by or dispensed from a pharmacy, the data from each transaction is entered and recorded in the computer. As long as all additions (quantities received) and subtractions (quantities dispensed or returned) from the inventory were entered correctly and accurately, the computer can generate a reliable inventory report at any given time.

What is an inventory report?
An inventory report is a detailed, itemized list that shows the quantity of each product the pharmacy has on-hand.

What is an override report?

When the actual on-hand quantity of a particular drug is different from the on-hand quantity recorded in the computer, a pharmacist or technician may manually change the number in the computer to match the actual on-hand quantity. Whenever the computer inventory numbers are manually changed, the computer automatically documents the details of the change and the identity of the person who made the change. Pharmacists and upper-level management can review this information at any time by generating an override report.

What is drug diversion?

Drug diversion is the act of obtaining medications for uses that are illegal or medically unauthorized. For instance, while filling a prescription for Percocet® (a narcotic pain medication), a pharmacy employee takes a tablet for her own personal use. This is a case of drug diversion. This employee will be fired and will likely suffer legal consequences for her actions.

What is a diversion report?

Similar to override reports, some pharmacy information systems are capable of generating diversion reports. These reports allow pharmacists and upper-level management to review pharmacy records that the computer flags as being potential cases of drug diversion.

What is eMAR?

Electronic medication administration (eMAR) programs are computerized systems that are used to maintain detailed records regarding administration of medications in an institutional setting (e.g. hospitals). For example, eMAR records typically include:

- The identity of the nurse who administered the medication.
- The identity of the patient who received the medication.
- The name and dose of medication administered.
- The date and time of administration.

Databases are frequently used by pharmacists and prescribers to find accurate information about medications quickly. Databases function almost like a search engine (e.g. Google, Yahoo, Bing), but the information contained in databases comes from manufacturers, research studies (e.g. clinical trial data), professional journals, and other reputable sources. Unlike the results of a basic internet search, the results of a database search are considered to be reliable.

Some common drug databases are listed below:
- Micromedex
- Drug Facts & Comparisons
- Gold Standard Drug Database
- Lexi-Comp
- Natural Medicines Comprehensive Database (for vitamins & supplements)

What information could you expect to find in a drug database?
- Available dosage forms of a particular drug
- Dosage form images and/or images of the packaging
- Mechanism of action
- Therapeutic dose ranges
- Overdose information
- Pharmacokinetics
- List of side effects
- Data from clinical studies
- Black box warnings
- Contraindications/cautions
- Safety/monitoring
- Storage instructions
- Patient education

Most drug databases also have useful applications, such as:
- Drug identifier
- Drug interaction checker
- IV drug compatibility checker
- Drug dose calculators

PTCB Certification
Renewal Requirements

Once you become PTCB certified, be aware that your certification must be renewed every 2 years. The recertification fee is $40. To be eligible for renewal, you must obtain 20 hours of continuing education (CE) every 2 years. Of the 20 hours of CE, at least 1 hour must be on the topic of pharmacy law and 1 hour on patient safety. All CE hours earned after January 1, 2015 must be in pharmacy technician-specific subject matter. For more information on PTCB certification renewal, see the PTCB website (PTCB.org).

Congratulations! You are almost prepared to take the PTCB exam. Before ending your study efforts, I would recommend that you review the math sections of this book a few more times, especially in the final week leading up to the exam. Being successful in solving math problems is crucial to your overall success on the exam. Once you are finished with this study guide, consider taking an Official PTCB Practice Exam, available online at <**https://app.testrac.com/ptcb/delivery/**>. The Official PTCB Practice Exam is $29. If you're not confident enough yet to spend $29 on the official practice exam, I recommend taking another practice exam available from *PTCB Exam Simplified*, which you can obtain for FREE (see page 275 for details).

Tips to help you perform well on the actual exam:
- If you have never been to the testing center where you scheduled your exam, drive there a day or two prior to the exam so you know how to get there.
- Ensure you are well-rested, well-hydrated, and well-fed on exam day.
- Do not rush through the exam; remain calm.
- The test is multiple-choice, so if you don't know the right answer to a question/problem, then try to eliminate some of the choices which you *know* are incorrect.
- When you don't know an answer and you are forced to guess, do not select an answer you have never heard of (e.g. if you have it narrowed down to: "A. Diabetes" or "B. Diffuse Intravascular Coagulation," then choose "A. Diabetes"). The answer is probably easier than you think.
- As previously mentioned, the entire exam is multiple-choice (including the math problems). Usually multiple-choice exams benefit the test-taker, but be careful! When math problems are presented in a multiple-choice format, the various choices are often designed to trick and deceive you. My advice for any question involving math is to do the problem and double check your answer using a calculator before you even look at any of the multiple-choice answer options. This prevents you from being influenced by the wrong answers.
- Remember, you will get 110 minutes to complete the PTCB exam and you will need to earn a scaled score of 650 to pass. That means you have to get about 70% of the questions correct. The practice exam in the pages that follow consists of 90 problems, just like the real PTCB exam. For the purposes of this practice exam, assume each problem is worth one point. For answers that are completely or partially wrong, you do not get the point. When you are finished, add up all of your points and divide that quantity by 90. You will get a decimal (something between 0.00 and 1.00). Multiply that number by 100%. For instance, if you answered 80 of the questions correctly, you would divide 80 by 90, which equals 0.89. So take 0.89 and multiply that by 100%. That equals 89%. An 89% would be an example of a passing score (> 70%).

Proceed with confidence!
-David

Practice Exam

1. Mrs. Tucker weighs 65 kg. What is Mrs. Tucker's weight in pounds?

    A. 65 lbs
    B. 130 lbs
    C. 143 lbs
    D. 150 lbs
    E. 156 lbs

2. If a bottle of Protonix® has a manufacturer-assigned expiration date of 09/2015, what is the last day it can be used?

    A. August 31, 2015
    B. September 1, 2015
    C. September 30, 2015
    D. October 1, 2015
    E. None of the above

3. What is the generic drug name for Keppra®?

    A. lansoprazole
    B. lamotrigine
    C. ipratropium
    D. levetiracetam
    E. levofloxacin

4. Which insulin formulation(s) is/are considered "rapid acting?"

    A. NovoLog®
    B. Levemir®
    C. Apidra®
    D. Both A and B.
    E. Both A and C.

5. By what routes can the antibiotic vancomycin be administered?

    A. Oral.
    B. Transdermal.
    C. Intravenous.
    D. Both A and C.
    E. All of the above.

6. Which drug class is associated with the side effect of a dry, nonproductive cough?

    A. Beta Blockers
    B. Angiotensin Receptor Blockers
    C. HMG-CoA Reductase Inhibitors
    D. Serotonin-Norepinephrine Reuptake Inhibitors
    E. Angiotensin Converting Enzyme Inhibitors

7. **A patient who takes Coumadin® is more likely to experience bleeding problems when taking which of these medications?** (select all that apply)

- ☐ aspirin
- ☐ naproxen
- ☐ Augmentin®
- ☐ ciprofloxacin
- ☐ clindamycin

8. **Match each brand name with the correct generic name.**

A. Lodine®	I. ketorolac
B. Tessalon®	II. citalopram
C. Dilantin®	III. etodolac
D. Valium®	IV. escitalopram
E. Toradol®	V. diazepam
F. Lexapro®	VI. benzonatate
G. Celexa®	VII. phenytoin
H. Desyrel®	VIII. trazodone
I. Singulair®	IX. terbinafine
J. Medrol®	X. methylprednisolone
K. Lamisil®	XI. Montelukast

9. **Match each drug with the condition that it can be used to treat.**

A. meloxicam	I. osteoporosis
B. fexofenadine	II. depression
C. oxybutynin	III. allergies
D. olmesartan	IV. inflammation
E. carbamazepine	V. insomnia
F. buspirone	VI. diabetes mellitus
G. fentanyl	VII. seizure disorders
H. zolpidem	VIII. hypertension
I. alendronate	IX. pain
J. exenatide	X. overactive bladder
K. bupropion	XI. anxiety

10. **Which of the following agencies is responsible for enforcing the Federal Controlled Substance Act?**

    A. FDA
    B. DEA
    C. OSHA
    D. FTC
    E. None of the above

11. **Which controlled substance schedule fits the following description?**
Contains drugs that are used medically, but have a high potential for abuse and physical/psychological dependence.

    A. Schedule I
    B. Schedule II
    C. Schedule III
    D. Schedule IV
    E. Schedule V

12. What is the name of the paper form used to order Schedule II controlled substances?

    A. DEA Form 41
    B. DEA Form 222
    C. Invoice
    D. DEA Form 106
    E. Pharmacy C-II Order Sheet

13. What is the purpose of the Health Insurance Portability and Accountability Act of 1996 (HIPAA)?

    A. To require drug utilization reviews for Medicaid patients.
    B. To protect children from serious injury from ingesting medications.
    C. To prevent the use of pseudoephedrine in illegal drug production.
    D. To require drug utilization reviews for Medicare Part D patients.
    E. To protect the privacy of patient health information.

14. The Poison Prevention Packaging Act (PPPA) is intended to prevent accidental deaths in which age group?

    A. 5 years and younger
    B. 4 years and younger
    C. 12 years and younger
    D. 8 years and younger
    E. 2 years and younger

15. What is the name of the REMS program for isotretinoin?

    A. T.I.P.S.
    B. S.T.E.P.S.
    C. iPLEDGE
    D. Clozaril National Registry
    E. The Isotretinoin Damage Prevention Program

16. What is the maximum amount of pseudoephedrine one person may purchase in one day?

    A. 2 grams
    B. 3.6 grams
    C. 7.5 grams
    D. 9 grams
    E. 5 boxes

17. Why is thalidomide available only through a restricted drug program?

    A. Thalidomide is known to cause cancer.
    B. Thalidomide is known to cause birth defects.
    C. Thalidomide is known to cause renal (kidney) failure.
    D. Thalidomide is associated with hypoglycemia.
    E. Thalidomide is a strong acid that causes duodenal ulcers.

18. In what order should the following clean room garb be donned? (arrange from first to last)

    ___ Shoe Covers
    ___ Gloves
    ___ Gown
    ___ Face Mask
    ___ Hair Cover

19. When filtering a Total Nutrient Admixture (TNA; which contains emulsified fat droplets), what pore size should the filter have?

    A. 1 centimeter
    B. 0.5 microns
    C. 0.22 microns
    D. 1.2 microns
    E. None of the above

20. What is wrong with the prescription shown below?

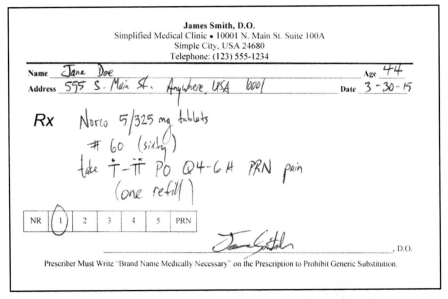

    A. Refills cannot be issued for a Schedule II controlled substance.
    B. The patient's state-issued ID number is not written on the prescription.
    C. The prescriber's DEA number is not written on the prescription.
    D. Both A & C.
    E. All of the above.

21. What is the correct days' supply and DAW code to use when billing the patient's insurance for the prescription shown in question #20?

    A. 15-day supply; DAW 9.
    B. 10-day supply; DAW 1.
    C. 8-day supply; DAW 0.
    D. 5-day supply; DAW 0.
    E. 7-day supply; DAW 0.

22. Which two substances are most likely to bind with calcium and form an insoluble precipitate?

    A. Vitamin C and phosphate
    B. Vitamin D and biotin
    C. Vitamin B6 and saw palmetto
    D. Vitamin A and atorvastatin
    E. Vitamin E and chlorine

23. You are in the clean room and an order comes in for norepinephrine 10 mg in 250 mL of D5W. How many vials of norepinephrine solution will you need to open to prepare this order if the norepinephrine comes in 4 mg/4 mL vials?

    A. 1 vial
    B. 2 vials
    C. 3 vials
    D. 4 vials
    E. 2.5 vials

24. You are using a class A prescription balance with a sensitivity requirement of 6 mg. Using this balance, you can measure 300 mg of a substance within ___ % error.

    A. 1
    B. 2
    C. 3
    D. 4
    E. 5

25. You receive an order for 90 mL of lidocaine 4% nasal spray. You will use normal saline solution and 10% lidocaine solution to compound this prescription. How much 10% lidocaine solution will be needed?

    A. 18 mL
    B. 27 mL
    C. 36 mL
    D. 45 mL
    E. 54 mL

26. A patient presents a prescription for 450 milliliters of allopurinol 40 mg/mL oral suspension. Allopurinol is available from the manufacturer in an oral tablet form only. Using allopurinol 100 mg tablets, how many tablets will you pulverize and triturate to compound this prescription?

     A. 90 tablets
     B. 100 tablets
     C. 125 tablets
     D. 180 tablets
     E. 250 tablets

27. Hydralazine and Hydroxyzine are examples of _____.

     A. Allergy medications
     B. Brand name medications
     C. Separating inventory
     D. Look-alike/sound-alike medications
     E. Drug regimen reviews

28. Humalog® and NovoLog® are examples of _____.

     A. Rapid acting Insulin
     B. Brand name medications
     C. High-alert medications
     D. All of the above
     E. None of the above

29. What is the purpose of tall man lettering?

     A. To emphasize the spelling differences between medications with similar names.
     B. To standardize the font size for medication names as they appear on stock bottles.
     C. To make it easier to separate inventory.
     D. To eliminate the need for NDC numbers.
     E. None of the above.

30. How does the use of leading zeros affect the likelihood of a prescription order interpretation error?

     A. Use of leading zeros increases the likelihood of an error.
     B. Use of leading zeros decreases the likelihood of an error.
     C. Use of leading zeros has no effect on the likelihood of an error.
     D. It depends on who the patient is.

31. Which situation requires pharmacist intervention?

    A. Taking a new prescription from a new patient.
    B. Answering the telephone.
    C. Counting the tablets to fill a prescription for amlodipine.
    D. Recommending an OTC medication for a patient.
    E. All of the above.

32. Why are anticoagulant medications, such as heparin, considered "high-alert" medications institutional settings (e.g. hospitals and long-term care facilities)?

    A. Because they have a caffeine-like effect.
    B. Because over 20% of patients are allergic to these medications.
    C. Because high doses can cause severe and potentially fatal bleeding.
    D. Because overdoses can cause hypoglycemia.

33. Which employee(s) is/are authorized to perform a drug utilization review (DUR)?

    A. Pharmacy Technician
    B. Certified Pharmacy Technician
    C. Pharmacist
    D. Cashier
    E. Both B. and C.

34. What two entities are working together in a campaign to eliminate the use of error-prone abbreviations?

    A. FDA and DEA
    B. FBI and CIA
    C. WHO and OSHA
    D. ISMP and FDA
    E. IRS and FDIC

35. For a physician to prescribe Suboxone® outside of a narcotic treatment facility, he/she must have a special DEA number that begins with which letter?

    A. A
    B. F
    C. X
    D. Y
    E. Z

36. Which of the following could be an example of an NDC number?

    A. 0093-0437-01
    B. 01232-543-1
    C. 9678-234-09
    D. 00781-5824-100
    E. All of the above

37. When handling needles (e.g. when compounding sterile products for infusion), it is important that you:

    A. Always recap the needle after it has been used.
    B. Never recap the needle after it has been used.
    C. Place the used needle in a red sharps container.
    D. Both A. and C.
    E. Both B. and C.

38. Which class of FDA recall would be issued for a product that is unlikely to cause any adverse health effects?

    A. Class I
    B. Class II
    C. Class III
    D. Class IV
    E. Class A

39. Which technologies helped improve the quality of healthcare delivery? (Select all that apply)

    ☐   Computerized Physician Order Entry (CPOE)
    ☐   E-Prescribing
    ☐   DAW Codes
    ☐   Bar-Code Technology
    ☐   Prior Authorizations

40. How many refills can a patient receive on a C-III medication, and for what length of time is the prescription valid (according to federal law)?

    A. 12 refills; 12 months
    B. 11 refills; 12 months
    C.5 refills; 6 months
    D. No refills; 30 days

41. Which statement best describes Provigil® (modafinil)?

    A. It is a non-controlled substance used for the treatment of diarrhea.
    B. It is a Schedule I controlled substance with no medically accepted uses.
    C. It is a Schedule IV controlled substance used to treat fatigue.
    D. It is a Schedule III controlled substance used to treat insomnia
    E. It is a Schedule V controlled substance used to treat opioid addiction.

42. On the prescription below, is the prescriber's DEA number valid?

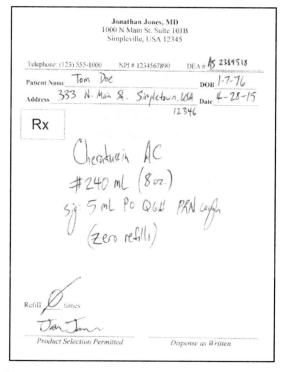

Jonathan Jones, MD
1000 N Main St. Suite 101B
Simpleville, USA 12345

Telephone: (123) 555-1000   NPI # 1234567890   DEA # AS 2389518

Patient Name Tom Doe   DOB 1-7-76

Address 333 N. Main St. Simpletown, USA   Date 4-28-15
12346

Rx

Cheratussin AC
#240 mL (8 oz.)
sig: 5 mL PO Q6H PRN cough
(zero refill)

Refill ___ times

Product Selection Permitted   Dispense as Written

A. Yes
B. No
C. Not enough information to answer the question

43. How many teaspoonsful are contained in 240 mL and what is the days' supply of Cheratussin® AC for the prescription from question #40?

A. 8 teaspoonsful; 12-day supply.
B. 8 teaspoonsful; 8-day supply.
C. 16 teaspoonsful; 12-day supply.
D. 48 teaspoonsful; 12-day supply.
E. 48 teaspoonsful; 8-day supply.

44. The drug prescribed in question #40 belongs to which of the following categories?

A. Non-controlled substance.
B. Schedule II controlled substance.
C. Schedule III controlled substance.
D. Schedule V controlled substance.
E. Both A & C.

45. Which of the following pieces of information is *most* useful in the event of a recall?

    A. UPC Code
    B. Expiration Date
    C. Lot Number
    D. Manufacturer Phone Number
    E. None of the above

46. Which reference would you use to find out if one drug product is therapeutically equivalent to another drug product?

    A. Lexi-Comp
    B. Gold Standard Drug Database
    C. Micromedex
    D. Orange Book
    E. Sunrise Pharmacy

47. If the manufacturer-assigned expiration date for a bottle of medication is 01/2019, after which of the following days will the contents of the bottle expire?

    A. January 1, 2018
    B. January 1, 2019
    C. January 15, 2019
    D. January 30, 2019
    E. January 31, 2019

48. If a prescriber writes a prescription for CCXL milliliters of Hydromet® oral solution, how many milliliters should you dispense?

    A. 8 ounces
    B. 120 mL
    C. 240 mL
    D. 360 mL
    E. 480 mL

49. According to the manufacturer, Travatan Z® eye drops should be stored at, or between, 2-25°C. Which of the following environments would be acceptable for storing Travatan Z®?

    A. A cold environment
    B. A cool environment
    C. A room temperature environment
    D. Both B. and C.
    E. All of the above

50. Which of the following programs could be used to maintain a patient's medication history?

    A. Meditech
    B. Micromedex
    C. The Orange Book
    D. Lexi-Comp
    E. Medicaid

51. A patient drops off a prescription for an 84-day supply of Trinessa®, but her insurance will only pay for a 28-day supply. This is an example of a _____.

    A. Coordination of benefits
    B. Refill to soon rejection
    C. Co-payment
    D. Prior authorization
    E. Plan limitation

52. Home infusion pharmacies specialize in dispensing what kind of products?

    A. Sterile infusion products
    B. Bioequivalent hormone replacement products
    C. Orally administered drug products
    D. Durable medical equipment
    E. Oxygen and medical supplies

53. Which parts of Medicare can be billed for prescription drugs?

    A. Part A
    B. Part B
    C. Part C
    D. Part D
    E. Both B. and D.

54. Sandra has prescription drug coverage through Insurance Company X, but she has never used it. Which of the following types of payments has Sandra probably made to Insurance Company X?

    A. Premium
    B. Deductible
    C. Co-payment
    D. All of the above
    E. None of the above

55. Who is responsible for the administration of Medicare?

    A. DEA
    B. FDA
    C. CMS
    D. ISMP
    E. President Obama

56. The pharmacist tells you that he wants the refrigerator temperature to be set to 6°C. What is this temperature in degrees Fahrenheit?

  A. 0°F
  B. 32°F
  C. 35°F
  D. 43°F
  E. 100°F

57. If a solution of ampicillin is being infused at the rate of 60 drops per minute, how long will it take to infuse 100 milliliters assuming that the administration set delivers 20 drops per milliliter?

  A. 23 minutes
  B. 25minutes
  C. 30 minutes
  D. 33 minutes
  E. 35 minutes

58. Tanya weighs 210 pounds and has a life-threatening fungal infection. Her physician prescribes a 0.3 mg/kg dose of amphotericin B. How many micrograms of amphotericin B should Tanya receive?

  A. 29 mg
  B. 63 mg
  C. 29,000 mcg
  D. 63,000 mcg
  E. 33 mg

59. The dose of experimental drug DH671244 is 55 mg/m² every 8 hours. How many milligrams of DH671244 should be given over the course of 24 hours for a male patient that is exactly 6 feet tall and weighs 240 pounds?

  A. 190 mg
  B. 280 mg
  C. 390 mg
  D. 460 mg
  E. 530 mg

60. **What is wrong with the way the following prescription is written?**

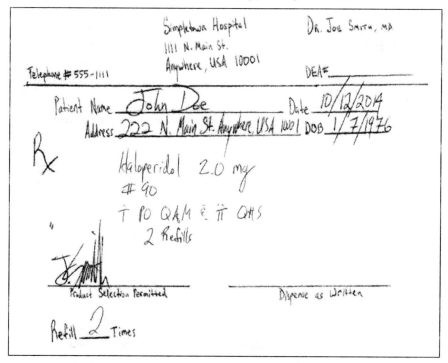

A. The insurance will not cover this medication for a 30-day supply.
B. The prescriber used a trailing zero.
C. The prescriber's DEA number is not written on the prescription.
D. The prescriber did not sign on the "Dispense as Written" line.
E. All of the above.

61. Approximately how many tablespoons comprise 2 ounces of a liquid?

A. 8 teaspoons
B. 4 teaspoons
C. 2 tablespoons
D. 4 tablespoons
E. ½ of a cup

62. Which of the following substances would be the most appropriate choice for cleaning a laminar airflow hood (LAFH)?

A. 70% isopropyl alcohol
B. 90% isopropyl alcohol
C. 70% ethyl alcohol
D. 90% ethyl alcohol
E. Windex®

63. Of the following choices, which controlled substance schedule has the highest potential for dependence and abuse?

    A. Schedule V
    B. Schedule IV
    C. Schedule III
    D. Schedule II
    E. All of the above

64. Which of the following medications is not used for treating depression?

    A. venlafaxine
    B. fluoxetine
    C. hydralazine
    D. mirtazepine
    E. escitalopram

65. Why type of dosage form must be shaken well prior to use?

    A. Elixir
    B. Solution
    C. Suspension
    D. Cream
    E. Ointment

66. Which statement is true regarding medications for the eye?

    A. Eye drops can be used in the ear.
    B. Ear drops can be used in the eye.
    C. Oral solutions can be used in the eye.
    D. Oral solutions can be used in the ear.
    E. Enemas can be used in the eye.

67. You are at a pharmacy that purchased 30-tablet bottles of clopidogrel 75 mg from their distributor at a WAC of $59.95. The pharmacist instructs you to set the retail price based on a markup of 12% and a dispensing fee of $11. A patient calls the pharmacy asking for the price of 60 tablets of clopidogrel 75 mg. The patient is not using insurance. Which response is correct?

    A. $78.14
    B. $145.29
    C. $156.29
    D. $176.14

68. How frequently must you renew your PTCB certification?

    A. Every year
    B. Every 2 years
    C. Every 3 years
    D. Every 4 years
    E. Every 5 years

69. What is the purpose of rotating stock?

    A. To ensure that patients are receiving the newest medication first.
    B. To reduce the profitability of the pharmacy.
    C. To decrease the emphasis on patient safety.
    D. To ensure that drugs closer to expiration are dispensed first.
    E. To maintain a clean and orderly appearance in the pharmacy.

70. Which of the following statements is correct regarding scored tablets?

    A. Scored tablets should never be split or cut.
    B. Scored tablets are designed for sublingual administration.
    C. Scored tablets always have a circular shape.
    D. Scored tablets are designed to be easily split into fractions.
    E. Scored tablets will not dissolve until they reach the small intestine.

71. Which of the following is a type of insurance plan?

    A. NDC
    B. PBM
    C. CMS
    D. PPE
    E. PPO

72. Which of the following patients is not allowed to use a manufacturer coupon for her Advair® prescription?

    A. Elizabeth, who is insured through her employer.
    B. Edith, who does not have prescription drug insurance.
    C. Sarah, who is enrolled in Medicaid.
    D. None of the above.

73. Which law requires patient counseling by a pharmacist?

    A. Health Insurance Portability and Accountability Act
    B. Poison Prevention Packaging Act
    C. Combat Methamphetamine Epidemic Act
    D. Comprehensive Drug Abuse Prevention and Control Act
    E. Omnibus Reconciliation Act

74. If the normal adult dose of clindamycin is 300 mg, then what is the dose for a 4 year old patient that weighs 60 pounds? (calculate the dose using Clark's Rule)

    A. 55 mg
    B. 100 mg
    C. 110 mg
    D. 120 mg
    E. 165 mg

75. Federal law indicates that prescription records must be kept for 2 years, but the state law where you work indicates that prescription records must be kept for 3 years. The records should be kept for _____.

    A. 2 years
    B. 2 & ½ years
    C. 3 years
    D. 4 years
    E. None of the above

76. A prescription is written for pednisone 10 mg tablets with instructions for the patient to take 4 tablets daily for 2 days, then 3 tablets daily for 2 days, then 2 tablets daily for 2 days, then 1 tablet daily for 2 days, then ½ tablet daily for 2 days, then stop. How many tablets will you need to dispense?

    A. 18 tablets
    B. 21 tablets
    C. 24 tablets
    D. 27 tablets
    E. 30 tablets

77. A prescription is written for 60 tablets of bupropion XL 150 mg with instructions for the patient to take 1 tablet by mouth once daily for 8 days and then take 2 tablets by mouth once daily thereafter. What is the days' supply for this prescription?

    A. 27 days
    B. 30 days
    C. 33 days
    D. 34 days
    E. 38 days

78. While preparing an IV admixture, you observe an unexpected color change. This is most likely a sign of _____.

    A. Expiration
    B. Adverse drug reaction
    C. Side effect
    D. Bacterial contamination
    E. Incompatibility

79. Which vitamin can be used to lower cholesterol and triglycerides?

A. Vitamin A (retinol)
B. Vitamin B1 (thiamine)
C. Vitamin C (ascorbic acid)
D. Vitamin B3 (niacin)
E. Vitamin D2 (ergocalciferol)

80. Which one of the following insulin formulations is available over-the-counter (OTC)?

A. Lantus
B. Novolin 70/30
C. Levemir
D. Humalog
E. Apidra

81. Which one of the following products reverses the effect of warfarin?

A. Vitamin K
B. Aspirin
C. Tylenol®
D. Senna
E. Metformin

82. Which of the following medications is typically considered a "high-alert medication?"

A. Citalopram
B. Metoprolol
C. Fluticasone
D. Heparin
E. Hydrocortisone

83. Which herbal supplement can be used to alleviate symptoms of menopause?

A. SAM-e
B. Melatonin
C. Witch Hazel
D. Black Cohosh
E. Red Yeast Rice

84. A 6 year old child needs to receive experimental drug AP22233, but there is no well-established pediatric dose. If the normal adult dose is 3 mg, what dose should this child receive based on Young's Rule?

    A. 0.33 mg
    B. 0.5 mg
    C. 0.67 mg
    D. 1 mg
    E. 1.33 mg

85. Which law gives the Food and Drug Administration authority to require manufacturers to comply with Risk Evaluation and Mitigation Strategies?

    A. FDA Amendments Act of 2007
    B. Omnibus Reconciliation Act of 1990
    C. Comprehensive Drug Abuse Prevention and Control Act
    D. Health Insurance Portability and Accountability Act of 1996
    E. Combat Methamphetamine Epidemic Act of 2005

86. Which of the following drug names is an example of a brand name?

    A. Albuterol HFA
    B. Lisinopril
    C. Naproxen
    D. Motrin
    E. Ibandronate

87. How many grams of each ingredient are needed to compound the prescription below?

Simpletown Hospital
1111 N. Main St.
Anywhere, USA 10001

Dr. Joe Smith, MD

Telephone # 555-1111

DEA#_____

Patient Name __John Doe__ Date 10/12/2014

Address 222 N. Main St. Anywhere, USA 1001 DOB 1/7/1976

℞

1:1 Mixture

Eucerin cream & Triamcinolone 0.5% oint.
Dispense: one pound jar
Sig: AAA BID PRN itchy rash
(NR)

Product Selection Permitted

Dispense as Written

Refill __0__ Times

A. 500 g Eucerin Cream & 500 g Triamcinolone 0.5% Ointment
B. 227 g Eucerin Cream & 227 g Triamcinolone 0.5% Ointment
C. 500 g Eucerin Cream & 500 g Triamcinolone 1% Ointment
D. 254 g Eucerin Cream & 254 g Triamcinolone 1% Ointment
E. 0.5 kg Eucerin Cream & 0.5 kg Triamcinolone 1% Ointment

88. How has Dr. Joe Smith implemented safety strategies for the bupropion prescription pictured below?

Simpletown Hospital
1111 N. Main St.
Anywhere, USA 10001

Dr. Joe Smith, MD

Telephone # 555-1111

DEA#_____

Patient Name John Doe   Date 10/12/2014
Address 222 N. Main St. Anywhere, USA 10001   DOB 1/7/1976

℞

BuPROPion XL 300 mg
30 tablets
take one tablet by mouth once daily.
2 Refills

_____Product Selection Permitted_____   _____Dispense as Written_____

Refill 2 Times

A. Dr. Smith used tall man lettering.
B. Dr. Smith did not use any error-prone abbreviations.
C. Dr. Smith did not use trailing zeros.
D. All of the above.

89. A patient presents a prescription for Clindamycin 300 mg capsules with instructions to take 300 mg by mouth every 6 hours for 14 days. How many capsules should you dispense?

A. 42 capsules
B. 56 capsules
C. 68 capsules
D. 72 capsules
E. Not enough information

90. What does the sig code AU stand for?

A. Left eye
B. Both eyes
C. Left ear
D. Both ears
E. Australia

PRACTICE EXAM
ANSWER KEY

1. C. 143 lbs

$$\frac{65\,kg}{1} \times \frac{2.2\,lbs}{kg} = 143\ lbs$$

2. C. September 30, 2015

    To review this topic, see "Lot Numbers and Expiration Dates" on page 213.

3. D. levetiracetam

Brand Name	Generic Name
Prevacid®	lansoprazole
Lamictal®	lamotrigine
Atrovent®	ipratropium
Keppra®	levetiracetam
Levaquin®	levofloxacin

4. E. Both A and C.

Category	Brand Name	Onset of Action	Duration of Action
Rapid Acting	Apidra®, Humalog®, NovoLog®	15 - 30 min.	3 - 6 hours
Short Acting	Humulin R®, Novolin R®	30 - 60 min.	6 - 10 hours
Intermediate Acting	Humulin N®, Novolin N®	1 - 2 hours	16 - 24 hours
Long Acting	Lantus®, Levemir®	1 - 2 hours	24 hours
Ultra Long Acting	Tresiba®	1 hour	24 - 40 hours

5. D. Both A and C.

    Vancomycin is available as a tablet/capsule for oral administration and a solution for intravenous administration. To review this information, see "The Top 238 Prescription Drugs" on pages 60 – 78. Even though it is possible that you could get a question like this on the PTCB exam, I do not recommend that you spend too much time memorizing these types of really small details unless you have several months set aside for studying.

6. E. Angiotensin Converting Enzyme Inhibitors

    20% of patients that use anACE inhibitor develop a dry, non-productive cough. To review this topic, see page 30.

7. All of them.

    All of these drugs are NSAIDs or antibiotics. When taken with wafarin, these drugs can increase the risk of bleeding. To review this topic, see page 88.

8.
A. Lodine®	–	III. etodolac
B. Tessalon®	–	VI. benzonatate
C. Dilantin®	–	VII. phenytoin
D. Valium®	–	V. diazepam
E. Toradol®	–	I. ketorolac
F. Lexapro®	–	IV. escitalopram
G. Celexa®	–	II. citalopram
H. Desyrel®	–	VIII. trazodone
I. Singulair®	–	XI. montelukast
J. Medrol®	–	X. methylprednisolone
K. Lamisil®	–	IX. terbinafine

9.
A. meloxicam	–	IV. inflammation
B. fexofenadine	–	III. allergies
C. oxybutynin	–	X. overactive bladder
D. olmesartan	–	VIII. hypertension
E. carbamazepine	–	VII. seizure disorders
F. buspirone	–	XI. anxiety
G. fentanyl	–	IX. pain
H. zolpidem	–	V. insomnia
I. alendronate	–	I. osteoporosis
J. exenatide	–	VI. diabetes mellitus
K. bupropion	–	II. depression

10. B. DEA

Agency	Role
FDA	Enforces drug manufacturing laws. Regulates prescription drug advertising and large-scale compounding.
DEA	Enforces the federal Controlled Substances Act (CSA). Classifies controlled substances.
OSHA	Enforces health and safety laws.
FTC	Regulates over-the-counter drug, medical device, cosmetic, and food advertising.

11. B. Schedule II

Schedule	Medical Uses	Abuse Potential	Dependence Potential
C-I	No	High	High
C-II	Yes	High	High
C-III	Yes	Moderate	Moderate-Low
C-IV	Yes	Mild	Mild
C-V	Yes	Low	Low

12.   B. DEA Form 222

Form	Purpose
DEA Form 41	To report to the DEA the destruction of controlled substances
DEA Form 106	To report to the DEA the theft or loss of controlled substances.
DEA Form 222	To order (or to document the transfer of) Schedule I or Schedule II controlled substances

To review this topic further, see "DEA Forms" on pages 110 – 111.

13.   E. To protect the privacy of patient health information.

To review this topic, see "Health Insurance Portability & Accountability Act (HIPAA)" on page 117.

14.   A. 5 years and younger

To review this topic, see "Poison Prevention Packaging Act" on page 115.

15.   C. iPLEDGE

REMS Program	Drug Affected
iPLEDGE	isotretinoin
THALIDOMID REMS	Thalidomid® (thalidomide)
T.I.P.S.	Tikosyn® (dofetilide)
Clozaril National Registry	Clozaril® (clozapine)

16.   B. 3.6 grams

An individual may purchase up to 3.6 grams of pseudoephedrine in one day, but not more than 9 grams in any 30-day period. If purchasing pseudoephedrine online, an individual is limited to 7.5 grams in any 30-day period.

17.   B. Thalidomide is known to cause birth defects.

Thalidomide can only be obtained through THALIDOMID REMS™ because the drug is known to cause severe birth defects when used by pregnant women. Thalidomide is also associated with dangerous blood clots.

18.　　 1 Shoe Covers
　　　　 2 Hair Cover
　　　　 3 Face Mask
　　　　 4 Gown
　　　　 5 Gloves

In general, you want to put on your clean room garb in the order of dirtiest to cleanest (shoes are assumed to be the dirtiest and washed hands are considered to be the cleanest).

19.　　 D. 1.2 microns

1.2 micron pores are large enough to allow the fat droplets to pass through the filter without clogging it. Smaller pores would be clogged easily by the fat droplets, and larger pores would allow harmful fungi and particles to pass. To review this topic, see pages 149 – 150.

20.　　 D. Both A & C.

All hydrocodone combination products were recently reclassified by the DEA from Schedule III to Schedule II (effective October 6, 2014). According to federal law, refills are prohibited for all Schedule II controlled substances. Additionally, all prescriptions for controlled substances must include the prescriber's DEA number. There are no federal laws or rules that require any type of patient identification number to appear on the face of a prescription.

21.　　 D. 5-day supply; DAW 0.

Since the prescriber signed on the line that says "Product Selection Permitted" and the patient did not request brand, the DAW code is "0." The days' supply should always be calculated under the assumption that the patient will use the maximum amount of medication in accordance with the prescribed instructions. In this case, the maximum amount is 2 tablets every 4 hours, or 12 tablets per day. Some simple math tells us how many days the prescription should last:

$$\frac{60 \text{ tablets}}{1} \times \frac{\text{day}}{12 \text{ tablets}} = 5 \text{ days}$$

See pages 193 – 196 to review days' supply calculations and pages 224 – 225 to review DAW codes.

22.　　 A. Vitamin C and phosphate

Over time, Vitamin C (also known as ascorbic acid) breaks down to a substance called oxalate, which readily binds to calcium and forms an insoluble precipitate. Phosphate also binds readily to calcium and forms a precipitate. To review this topic, see page 150.

23.   C. 3 vials

The solution to this problem is unit conversion with a tricky twist. You
know that 10 mg of norepinephrine are needed to prepare the order, and
one vial contains 4 mg of norepinephrine. You will need a volume equal
to 2.5 vials to prepare the order; however, the question asks how many
vials you would need to *puncture/open* to prepare this order. You would
need to open 3 vials to obtain that volume. When taking the official PTCB
exam, pay close attention to the way each question is worded. Some of the
questions may be trickier than they first appear.

$$\frac{10\,mg}{1} \times \frac{vial}{4\,mg} = 2.5\,vials \therefore 3\,vials$$

24.   B. 2

If you know the sensitivity requirement of the balance (6 mg in this case)
and the weight of a substance being measured (300 mg), you can calculate
the percent error using the following equation:

$$\%\,Error = \frac{Sensitivity\ Requirement}{Measured Weight} \times 100\% = \frac{6\,mg}{300\,mg} \times 100\% = 2\%$$

25.   C. 36 mL

This is an alligation problem.

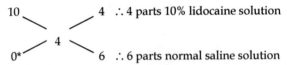

10   4   ∴ 4 parts 10% lidocaine solution

4

0*   6   ∴ 6 parts normal saline solution

<u>Note</u>: normal saline solution contains zero percent lidocaine.

This compound will consist of 10 parts (4 parts 10 % lidocaine solution
and 6 parts normal saline solution). In other words, four-tenths (4/10) of
the 90 mL prescription will be composed of the 10% lidocaine solution
and the other six-tenths (6/10) will be composed of normal saline solution
(i.e. 0% lidocaine solution).

$$\frac{90\,mL}{10\ parts} \times \frac{4\ parts\ of\ 10\%\ lidocaine}{1} = 36\,mL\,of\ 10\%\ lidociane$$

To review alligation, see pages 139 – 143.

26.   D. 180 tablets

To solve this problem, the first thing you must do is determine how many milligrams of allopurinol are needed to compound the entire prescription. This is a simple, one-step multiplication problem:

$$\frac{450\,\text{mL}}{1} \times \frac{40\,\text{mg}}{\text{mL}} = 18,000\,\text{mg}$$

Since we know there are 100 milligrams of allopurinol in each tablet, the next step is just as easy:

$$\frac{18,000\,\text{mg}}{1} \times \frac{\text{tablet}}{100\,\text{mg}} = 180\,\text{tablets}$$

27.   D. Look-alike/sound-alike medications.

To review look-alike/sound-alike medications, see page 159.

28.   D. All of the above

To review these topics, see pages 47 and 164.

29.   A. To emphasize the spelling differences between medications with similar names.

To review this topic, see page 160.

30.   B. Use of leading zeros decreases the likelihood of an error.

To review this topic, see page 161.

31.   D. Recommending an OTC medication for a patient.

To review situations requiring pharmacist intervention, see page 165.

32.   C. Because high doses can cause severe and potentially fatal bleeding.

To review the topic of high-alert medications, see page 164.

33.   C. Pharmacist

To review situations requiring pharmacist intervention, see page 165.

34.   D. ISMP and FDA

To review this point, see page 162.

35.   **C. X**

A unique DEA registration number that begins with an "X" is granted to prescribers who have obtained the necessary waiver* from the DEA to prescribe, administer, and/or dispense C-III through C-V controlled substances outside of a narcotic treatment facility for the treatment of narcotic addiction. For more on this topic, see page 108.

36.   **A. 0093-0437-01**

NDC numbers consist of 11 digits (a 5-digit segment to identify the manufacturer, a 4-digit segment to identify the drug product, and a 2-digit segment that is usually used to identify the package size). In some cases, when a segment contains one or more trailing zeros, a trailing zero will be omitted. For instance, 00093-0437-01 could be expressed in any one of the following three ways:

0093-0437-01
00093-437-01
00093-0437-1

37.   **E. Both B. and C.**

It is never a good idea to recap a needle. Recapping increases the chance of a needle stick injury. Red sharps containers are the standard waste disposal containers for medical needles and sharp objects.

38.   **C. Class III**

There are 3 classes of FDA recalls: Class I, Class II, and Class III. The class I recall is the most severe; in these cases, serious adverse health consequences, up to and including death, are possible. The class III recall is the least severe; in these cases, the recalled product is unlikely to cause any adverse health consequences.

39.   The following 3 options should have been selected:
- ☐ Computerized Physician Order Entry (CPOE)
- ☐ E-Prescribing
- ☐ Bar-Code Technology

Prior Authorizations and DAW Codes are related to insurance claims, not technologies that improve the quality of healthcare.

40.   **C. 5 refills; 6 months**

The federal Controlled Substances Act limits the amount of refills on Schedule III and IV controlled substance prescriptions to a maximum of 5 refills within 6 months.

41.   C. It is a Schedule IV controlled substance used to treat fatigue.

To review details about Provigil® (modafinil), see page 78.

42.   B. No

When asked whether or not a DEA number is valid, you are expected to apply the 4-step process outlined on page 113. When you take the DEA number shown on the prescription (AS2389518) and apply the 4 step verification process, you see that the last digit of the DEA number should be "1;" however, the last digit of this prescriber's DEA number is "8."

43.   D. 48 teaspoonsful; 12-day supply.

This is a 2-part question. The solution to the first part involves simple unit conversion (convert milliliters to teaspoons). If you got this part wrong, go back to the section titled "The Secret to Solving Nearly Any Pharmacy Math Problem," memorize the list of **Must-Know Conversion Factors,** and then practice solving problems using conversion factors. The second part of this problem is a days' supply calculation (see below). If you got the wrong answer for this part, go back and review the section titled "Days' Supply Calculations."

$$\frac{240\,mL}{1} \times \frac{dose}{5\,mL} \times \frac{day}{4\,doses} = 12 \text{ days}$$

44.   D. Schedule V controlled substance.

A medication is categorized as either C-I, C-II, C-III, C-IV, C-V, or non-controlled. There is no way to know which schedule a medication belongs to other than memorization. To review controlled substances, see pages 101 – 104.

45.   C. Lot Number

To review the topic of lot numbers, see page 213.

46.   D. Orange Book

To review the topic of therapeutic equivalence, see page 96.

47.   E. January 31, 2019

To review the topic of xxpiration dates, see page 213.

48.   C. 240 mL

CCXL is the Roman numeral form of the number 240. Although choice "A" (8 ounces) is equivalent to 240 mL, the question specifically asks how many *milliliters* should be dispensed. To review Roman numerals, see pages 181 – 182.

49.   E. All of the above

Temperature Ranges	
Cold	2°C to 8°C (36°F to 46°F)
Cool	8°C to 15°C (46°F to 59°F)
Room Temperature	20°C to 25°C (68°F to 77°F)

All of these environments fall within the manufacturer's recommended range of storage temperatures.

50.   A. Meditech

To review pharmacy information systems, see page 228.

51.   E. Plan limitation

To review the topic of insurance, see pages 219 – 223.

52.   A. Sterile infusion products

To review, see page 223.

53.   E. Both B. and D.

Typically pharmacies bill Medicare Part D, but in some cases Part B can be billed. See page 220 for more details.

54.   A. Premium

Since Sandra has coverage, we know that a premium is being paid. Deductibles and co-payments are only paid when the insurance is used. Since she has never used her insurance, we know she has never paid a deductible or co-payment. To review the topic of insurance, see pages 219 – 223.

55.   C. CMS

For more information on CMS, see page 220.

56.   D. 43°F

$$^{0}F = \left(\frac{9}{5} \times {}^{0}C\right) + 32$$

57.   D. 33 minutes

$$\frac{100\,mL}{1} \times \frac{20\,drops}{mL} \times \frac{minute}{60\,drops} = 33\,minutes$$

58.　　C. 29,000 mcg

Pay close attention to the units. This question specifically asked for an answer in micrograms.

$$\frac{210\,lbs}{1} \times \frac{kg}{2.2\,lbs} \times \frac{0.3\,mg}{kg} \times \frac{1,000\,mcg}{mg} = 28,636\,mcg \therefore 29,000\,mcg$$

59.　　C. 390 mg

The solution to this problem involves multiple steps. First, you need to calculate the patient's body surface area (BSA). To calculate BSA, you must convert height to centimeters and weight to kilograms. Once you determine the patient's BSA, multiply it by 55 mg/m² to calculate the dose. Finally, you must multiply the dose by 3 since the patient will receive 1 dose every 8 hours and the question asks how many milligrams will be given in a 24-hour period.

60.　　B. The prescriber used a trailing zero.

Use of trailing zeros could lead to interpretation errors; for example, 2 mg written as 2.0 mg could be misinterpreted as 20 mg.

61.　　D. 4 tablespoons

$$\frac{2\,ounces}{1} \times \frac{30\,mL}{ounce} \times \frac{1\,tablespoon}{15\,mL} = 4\,tablespoons$$

62.　　A. 70% isopropyl alcohol

To review this topic, see pages 144 – 152.

63.　　D. Schedule II

Schedule	Medical Uses	Abuse Potential	Dependence Potential
C-II	Yes	High	High
C-III	Yes	Moderate	Moderate-Low
C-IV	Yes	Mild	Mild
C-V	Yes	Low	Low

64.　　C. hydralazine

Hydralazine is a vasodilator used for the treatment of angina.

65.　　C. Suspension

To review, see the illustration on page 93.

66.   A. Eye drops can be used in the ear.

To review this topic, see page 166.

67.   B. $145.29

Retail Cost = WAC + Markup + Dispensing Fee

$$\text{Retail Cost} = \left(\frac{\$59.95}{bottle} \times 2\,bottles \right) + \left(\left(\frac{\$59.95}{bottle} \times 2\,bottles \right) \times 0.12 \right) + \$11 = \$145.29$$

<u>Note</u>: A dispensing fee is charged on a per prescription basis. This fee does not increase or decrease based on the quantity dispensed.

68.   B. Every 2 years

To review PTCB certification renewal, see page 232.

69.   D. To ensure that drugs closer to expiration are dispensed first.

To review this topc, see page 214.

70.   D. Scored tablets are designed to be easily split into fractions.

To review this topic, see page 94.

71.   E. PPO

To review the topic of insurance, see pages 219 – 223.

72.   C. Sarah, who is enrolled in Medicaid.

Prescription drug coupons cannot be used by individuals who are enrolled in a government prescription drug insurance program.

73.   E. Omnibus Reconciliation Act

To review this topic, see page 116.

74.   D. 120 mg

$$\text{Child dose} = \frac{60\,lbs}{150\,lbs} \times 300\,mg = 120 \text{ mg}$$

To review pediatric dosing equations, see pages 206 – 208.

75.   C. 3 years

You do not need to know specific state laws for the PTCB exam, but you do need to know that when federal and state laws differ, you must follow the more stringent law.

76.   B. 21 tablets

$$\left(\frac{4\,\text{tablets}}{\text{day}} \times 2\,\text{days}\right) + \left(\frac{3\,\text{tablets}}{\text{day}} \times 2\,\text{days}\right) + \left(\frac{2\,\text{tablets}}{\text{day}} \times 2\,\text{days}\right)$$
$$+ \left(\frac{1\,\text{tablet}}{\text{day}} \times 2\,\text{days}\right) + \left(\frac{0.5\,\text{tablet}}{\text{day}} \times 2\,\text{days}\right) = 21\,\text{tablets}$$

77.   D. 34 days

After the first 8 days of therapy, the patient will have 52 tablets remaining. Those 52 tablets will be sufficient to last 26 days (52 divided by 2, since the patient takes 2 tablets daily; see math below). So, the first 8 tablets last 8 days and the remaining 52 tablets will last 26 days. Then it is simple addition, 8 days + 26 days = 34 days.

$$\textit{For the first 8 days:} \ 8\,\text{tablets} \times \frac{\text{day}}{1\,\text{tablet}} = 8\,\text{days}$$

$$\textit{After the first 8 days:} \ 52\,\text{tablets} \times \frac{\text{day}}{2\,\text{tablets}} = 26\,\text{days}$$

78.   E. Incompatibility

To review the signs of incompatibility, see page 152.

79.   D. Vitamin B3 (niacin)

To review this topic, see pages 81 – 83.

80.   B. Novolin 70/30

****

Insulin Formulations Available Without a Prescription (OTC)

| Novolin N | Novolin R | Novolin 70/30 |
| Humulin N | Humulin R | Humulin 70/30 |

****

81.   A. Vitamin K

To review how warfarin works, see page 88.

82.   D. Heparin

To review high-alert medications, see page 164.

83.   D. Black Cohosh

To review the top 30 herbal supplements, see page 84.

84.   D. 1 mg

$$\text{Child Dose} = \frac{6}{(6+12)} \times 3\,\text{mg} = 1\,\text{mg}$$

To review pediatric dosing equations, see pages 206 – 208.

85.   A. FDA Amendments Act of 2007

To review Risk Evaluation and Mitigation Strategies, see pages 123 – 124.

86.   D. Motrin

Brand Name	Generic Name
ProAir®, Ventolin®, Proventil®	Albuterol HFA
Prinivil®, Zestril	Lisinopril
Aleve®, Naprosyn®	Naproxen
Motrin®, Advil®	Ibuprofen
Boniva®	Ibandronate

87.   B. 227 g Eucerin Cream & 227 g Triamcinolone 0.5% Ointment.

The prescription asks for a one pound mixture containing equal parts of Eucerin Cream and Triamcinolone 0.5% Ointment. This is a simple unit conversion problem. We already know that we need one-half pound of each ingredient. The question is: how many grams are in one-half pound? You must have the conversion factor committed to memory; there are 454 grams in 1 pound. One-half of 454 grams is 227 grams. So, to compound this prescription you will need 227 grams of Eucerin Cream and 227 grams of Triamcinolone 0.5% Ointment. If your answer was incorrect, you need to go back to page 185 and memorize the list of Must-Know Conversion Factors.

88.   D. All of the above.

To review safety strategies, see pages 160 – 163.

89.   B. 56 capsules

$$\frac{1\,\text{capsule}}{6\,\text{hours}} \times \frac{24\,\text{hours}}{\text{day}} \times \frac{14\,\text{days}}{1} = 54 \text{ capsules}$$

90.   D. Both ears

Sig Code	Meaning
AD	right ear
AS	left ear
AU	both ears
OD	right eye
OS	left eye
OU	both eyes

To review more sig codes, see pages 175-177.

$$\% \ \text{Error} = \frac{\text{Sensitivity Requirement}}{\text{Desired Weight}} \times 100\%$$

$$\text{Density} = \frac{\text{Mass}}{\text{Volume}}$$

$$\text{Specific Gravity} = \frac{\text{Density of Substance}}{\text{Density of Reference Substance}}$$

$$^{\circ}C = \frac{5}{9}(^{\circ}F - 32) \qquad\qquad ^{\circ}F = \left(\frac{9}{5} \times {}^{\circ}C\right) + 32$$

$$\text{BSA} = \sqrt{\frac{\text{height (cm)} \times \text{weight (kg)}}{3,600}}$$

$$\text{Child Dose (Clark's Rule)} = \frac{\text{Child's Weight (lbs)}}{150 \ \text{lbs}} \times \text{Adult Dose}$$

$$\text{Child Dose (Young's Rule)} = \frac{\text{Child's Age}}{(\text{Child's Age} + 12)} \times \text{Adult Dose}$$

$$\text{Child Dose (BSA Dosing)} = \frac{\text{Child's BSA}}{1.73 \ \text{m}^2} \times \text{Adult Dose}$$

FREE BONUS!

Our goal is to exceed your expectations, and that is why we are giving you an additional full-length practice exam (a $5.95 value) for FREE!* Just follow the instructions below to get your free practice exam!

Instructions:

1. Visit our website, www.RxStudyGuides.com
2. Purchase the Bonus Pracice Exam using coupon code FREE4ME
3. Receive a link in your e-mail to download the Bonus Practice Exam for free!

*This offer may be changed or canceled at any time without notice.

WE ARE COMMITTED TO QUALITY. IF YOU DISCOVER ANY ERRORS IN THIS STUDY GUIDE, PLEASE REPORT THEM AT YOUR EARLIEST CONVENIENCE TO ErrorReporting@RxStudyGuides.com

THANK YOU FOR CHOOSING PTCB EXAM SIMPLIFIED!